The Mentally
Impaired Elderly:
Strategies and Interventions
to Maintain Function

The Mentally Impaired Elderly: Strategies and Interventions to Maintain Function

Ellen D. Taira
Editor

The Haworth Press
New York • London • Sydney

The Mentally Impaired Elderly: Strategies and Interventions to Maintain Function has also been published as *Physical & Occupational Therapy in Geriatrics*, Volume 9, Numbers 3/4 1991.

The Haworth Press, Inc., 10 Alice Street, Binghamton, NY 13904-1580
EUROSPAN/Haworth, 3 Henrietta Street, London WC2E 8LU England
ASTAM/Haworth, 162-168 Parramatta Road, Stanmore, Sydney, N.S.W. 2048 Australia

Library of Congress Cataloging-in-Publication Data

The Mentally impaired elderly : strategies and interventions to maintain function / Ellen D. Taira, editor.
    p. cm.
    An update to: Therapeutic interventions for the person with dementia.
    "Has also been published as Physical & occupational therapy in geriatrics, v. 9, no. 3/4, 1991" – T.p. verso.
    Includes bibliographical references.
    ISBN 1-56024-168-3 (alk. paper)
    1. Alzheimer's disease – Treatment. 2. Senile dementia – Treatment. 3. Alzheimer's disease – Patients – Care. 4. Senile dementia – Patients – Care. I. Taira, Ellen D. II. Therapeutic interventions for the person with dementia.
    [DNLM: 1. Activities of Daily Living – in old age. 2. Dementia – rehabilitation. 3. Self Care – in old age. W1 PH683M v. 9 no. 3/4 / WM 220 M549]
RC523.M46 1991
618.97'683 – dc20
DNLM/DLC
for Library of Congress
                                     91-20816
                                         CIP

The Mentally Impaired Elderly: Strategies and Interventions to Maintain Function

CONTENTS

**Effects of a Multi-Strategy Program Upon Elderly
with Organic Brain Syndrome** 131
*Velma Russ Reichenbach, MAMS, OTR/L
Margaret M. Kirchman, PhD, OTR/L,
FAOTA*

**Program Planning in Geriatric Psychiatry: A Model
for Psychosocial Rehabilitation** 153
*Danielle N. Butin, OTR, MPH
Colleen Heaney, BS, MA*

ABOUT THE EDITOR

Ellen Dunleavey Taira, OTR, MPH, is affiliated with New York University Medical Center as Assistant Director of Restorative Services at Goldwater Memorial Hospital, a 900-bed, chronic-care facility. Throughout her career, she has provided her expertise, as an occupational therapist and a gerontologist, in a variety of community and institutional settings. Ms. Taira has worked as a case manager and researcher in a home health and day health program in San Francisco to provide background research in the support of expanded Medicare benefits. In her work as a program specialist in long-term care for the state of Hawaii, she assisted in the development of programs to serve the socially and economically needy elderly, compiled the first directory of long term care services in Hawaii, and promoted the integration of services for the disabled and the elderly.

Ms. Taira has served on numerous boards and committees to expand community-based services. She has written extensively on the subject of long term care, presented papers at professional conferences and seminars, and acted as spokesperson for the needs of the elderly disabled in many settings.

Introduction
Ellen D. Taira

This volume is about caring for the most vulnerable elderly, those with mental impairment. It is also an update of *Therapeutic Interventions for the Person with Dementia*, published in 1986, which focused on shedding a more positive light on treatment approaches. Five years ago there were fewer voices speaking of treatment. The climate of negativity created anxiety and fear in families, older persons and providers. Although the atmosphere of 'therapeutic nihilism' (Mace, 1986) is less apparent in the current literature fear and discouragement continue to pervade the thinking of many policy makers when planning long term care for the mentally impaired.

Of even greater concern is the tremendous number of mentally impaired older persons predicted to need care in the next century. In a sample of well, working class, white persons over 65 a federally financed study conducted in East Boston by Harvard Medical School researchers found that 10.3% had memory impairments or other mental problems and an astonishing 47.2 percent of persons over 85 in this group probably had Alzheimers (Evans, 1989). Amazingly, as this issue demonstrates, there is some cause for optimism as interventions to delay the loss of function in the mentally impaired older person are identified.

Older persons who are physically disabled but cognitively intact are less likely to be institutionalized and more able to put together an array of services with the help of friends, family and service providers, largely because they can articulate their wishes. The client as self advocate and person capable of decision making is partic-

1

ularly important in the face of life extending technology. With the new OBRA requirements the decisional capacity of adults has been reinforced and the need to honor their wishes made more specific.

The mentally impaired, in contrast, have fewer medical needs, are less able to advocate for themselves, and are less desirable nursing home candidates since reimbursement is lower for the ambulatory person. Yet care needs are often greater because persons with cognitive impairment need to be supervised in daily living activities, sometimes continually.

Despite many efforts to identify stages of Alzheimer's disease there remains considerable disagreement as to what to expect at different levels of impairment. Hence the focus in this issue on INTERVENTION and MAINTAINING FUNCTION. Writers address what works and doesn't work. There is important research on the role of temporal adaptation in self care and in a similar vein, relationship between apraxia and dressing skills (see Massey and Mitchell, Edwards et al.). For the person who is institutionalized, Reichenbach and Kirchman offer a very positive view of efforts to enrich the daily lives of residents using program enhancement.

The principle focus of most articles, however, whether directly or indirectly, is the environment, including the essential role of the caregiver in providing a safe place that promotes and enhances function and minimizes weaknesses and limitations. Reducing the amount of assistance provided by the caregiver is essential to affect cost savings. An older person who can manage toileting in a structured familiar environment will instantly lose this essential self care skill when faced with long corridors, unfamiliar rooms and the absence of a caregiver familiar with his or her own routine.

The collection begins with a theoretical model proposed by Corcoran and Gitlin which provides a framework that all of us providing care can use. The steps are simple, clear and easily applied to the information that follows. The case study offers hope and encouragement to carry us forward in the task of caring, as do all the selections in this very special and timely volume.

Your suggestions and recommendations are always welcome.

REFERENCES

Evans, D. et al., Prevalence of Alzheimer's Disease in Community Based Elderly. J Am Med Assoc, Nov 10, 89.

Mace, N., Home and Community Services for Alzheimer's Disease in *Therapeutic Interventions for the Person with Dementia*, Taira, E., ed. 1986.

Environmental Influences
on Behavior of the Elderly with Dementia:
Principles for Intervention in the Home

Mary Corcoran, MA, OTR/L
Laura N. Gitlin, PhD

SUMMARY. Individuals with Alzheimer's disease are likely to experience heightened sensitivity to influences from the environment. Such influences may contribute to a range of behaviors which may be maladaptive and pose difficulty for the caregiver. In order to understand and modify transactions between impaired individuals and the environment, an environmental model, developed by Barris and colleagues, is presented and expanded. From this discussion, twelve intervention principles are derived which can be used by a range of health care professionals to guide treatment. Case material exemplifies use of the twelve intervention principles.

INTRODUCTION

An emerging trend in health care today is the design of environments to enhance personal competence of special populations of older adults and specifically of those with diminished mental capacity or dementia (Institute of Medicine, 1988). The focus on environment for therapeutic intervention is based on an evolving literature which indicates the effectiveness of manipulating the physical and

Mary Corcoran is Assistant Professor and Laura N. Gitlin is Assistant Professor and Research Coordinator at Thomas Jefferson University, Department of Occupational Therapy, College of Allied Health Sciences.

This paper was supported in part by funds from the American Occupational Therapy Foundation and TirLawyn Geriatric Consortium.

Special thanks to Paul Wolpe, PhD, Department of Psychiatry, Thomas Jefferson University for his guidance.

social environment to enhance competence or reinforce residual memory and abilities of the elderly with dementia. Studies of institutionalized elderly with dementia disclose that frequency and severity of problem behaviors are reduced by matching environmental characteristics with individual capacities (Corcoran and Barrett, 1986; Dawson et al., 1986; Hall and Buckwalter, 1987; Hiatt, 1987; Rogers et al., 1987). State-of-the-art architectural design in institutions appears to minimize common problem behaviors such as wandering, agitation, and restlessness (Cohen and Crook, 1989). In the home setting, simple techniques, which include labeling commonly used household objects or pre-packaging clothing according to daily needs, are effective strategies to maintain a level of competence in the home for the older adult with dementia (Mace and Rabins, 1981; Rogers et al., 1987).

Although such environmental solutions have emerged in part from a broad ecology of aging perspective (Lawton and Nahemow, 1973; Lawton, 1989), specification of a framework to understand dimensions of household environments which influence behavior is lacking. An elaboration of an environmental framework is compelling for two primary reasons. First, families provide close to 90% of the primary care for the elderly with dementia in the home over the course of illness (Stone, Cafferata and Sangl, 1987; Special Committee on Aging, 1987; Select Committee on Aging, 1990). Also, recent research using qualitative methodology indicates that caregivers express a need to enhance their skills in providing effective care (Hasselkus, 1988). Nevertheless, informal caregivers have not traditionally received skill training in adapting the physical and social dimensions of the home to modify care management problems and optimize behavioral outcomes. Second, although need for the provision of a range of supportive services is recognized, caregivers continue to be an underserved population within the health care industry. The specificity of an environmental framework is critical for the development and implementation of therapeutic interventions which are theory-based and delivered in the home. Theory-based interventions have been identified as a critical need by both the research and clinical community (Gallagher, 1985; Abels, 1990).

The purpose of this paper is to present and expand an environmental framework initially formulated by Barris and colleagues (1985) in the field of occupational therapy. The discussion extends the original model to include specific environmental considerations which are significant for the elderly population with dementia and their caregivers. Case material based on funded research projects (sponsored by the TirLawyn Geriatric Consortium and the American Occupational Therapy Foundation), illustrates effective intervention strategies stemming from the proposed perspective. This framework serves as a basis for health practitioners and service providers to understand behavior of the elderly with dementia in such diverse settings as adult day care, nursing homes or day hospital programs.

DESCRIPTION OF THE MODEL

Building on the work of Lawton and others (Lawton, 1983; Lawton and Nahemow, 1973), Barris and colleagues conceive of environment as a hierarchy arranged in four concentric circles (see Figure 1). Each layer of the environment is characterized by distinct attributes which can be manipulated or modified to achieve a behavioral goal.

Arousal and press are critical concepts to the understanding of the link between person-environment and behavioral outcomes. Arousal refers to an internal state of an organism, with physiological and subjective manifestations influencing choice of behavior (Barris et al., 1985). Choices about behavior are also made based on the press of environment or expectations for certain behavior which stem from the setting (Lawton and Nahemow, 1973; Lawton, 1989). A high level of personal competence will increase ability to adapt to environments with varying degrees of press, whereas reduced competence leads to vulnerability to environmental influences and the potential for maladaptive behavioral outcomes (Lawton and Nahemow, 1973; Oakley, 1987). Adaptation is the process of maintaining relative equilibrium between personal competence and environmental demands (Rogers et al., 1987) and requires constant adjustment and modification. In the case of dementia, the challenge is to adjust arousal and press through manipulation of the dimensions of the environment to minimize expectations for behav-

FIGURE 1. Model of the Environment

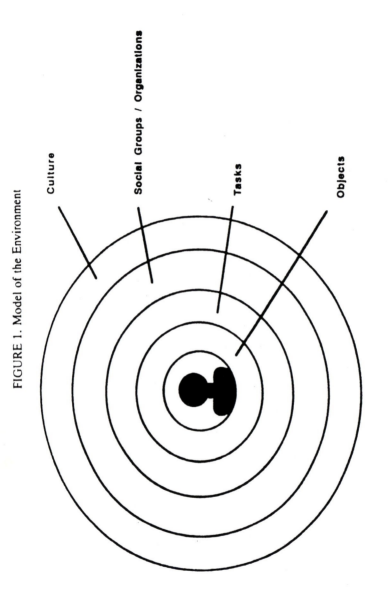

Culture

Social Groups / Organizations

Tasks

Objects

Barris et al. "Occupation as Interaction with the Environment.", A model of Human Occupation, 1975.

iors unavailable to the individual. In turn, environmental manipulation may maximize expectations for behaviors which may still be part of the individual's behavioral repertoire. As Lawton (1989) has argued there is perhaps no level of competence which is too low to respond positively to alterations in press.

The following discussion presents the meaning of each environmental layer and its dimensions and outlines principles for maintaining congruence or a fit between individuals with dementia and their environment or, a balance between competence and press (Lawton and Nahemow, 1973; Lawton, 1989).

OBJECT LAYER

The most inner layer and basic environmental category refers to objects or the physical materials which compose everyday life. Barris et al. identify four dimensions which contribute to the overall arousal and press of objects in the environment: availability, flexibility, complexity and symbolic meaning (Barris et al., 1985). These dimensions may have an independent or joint effect on behavior.

A. Availability

Availability refers to the degree of accessibility of objects in the environment. Researchers have noted that frail elderly often tend to centralize their living space by creating "control centers" which contain objects required for specific tasks or sets of tasks (Lawton, Brody and Saperstein, 1989; Rubinstein, 1989). The availability of necessary objects within a prescribed location provides an increased sense of control and ability to manipulate the immediate environment to achieve behavioral goals. In regard to the elderly with dementia, objects must not only be available but visually apparent in order to be utilized (Levy, 1987).

In contrast, decreasing an object's visibility may also heighten functional capacity of an individual with dementia. For example, putting away unnecessary clothing and shoes may assist in encouraging appropriate dress. *The first intervention principle that can be derived is that manipulation of degree of object availability may modify environmental press and in this way maintain or improve an individual's competence.*

B. Complexity

The second dimension, complexity, refers to the degree of skill and learning required for use of an object (Barris et al., 1985). An optimal environment for a person with dementia consists of highly familiar objects and surroundings. With limited short term memory, learning becomes unlikely early in the disease course (Levy, 1987; Oakley, 1987). Consequently, when a change in the environment is introduced which requires attaching a functional meaning to a previously unfamiliar or unknown object, a person with dementia may be at a loss.

Another aspect of complexity is the degree of difficulty in accessing way-finding cues from the overall environment. Calkins defines way-finding as an environmental process by which cues to aid navigation are obtained (Calkins, 1989). Information presented using diverse sensory pathways provides multiple cues to orientation. For example, apartment buildings designed especially for the elderly combine multiple cues in the elevator and floors to assure easy identification (Institute of Medicine, 1988). A person with dementia will benefit from strategies such as leaving lights on in key rooms (such as the bathroom) or labeling areas of the home with pictures of their primary function.

Removal of clutter also serves to highlight available way-finding cues (Hiatt, 1982). Clutter is defined as sensory input residual to or in excess of the intended task. Any sensory cue may be considered clutter if it presents confusion of stimuli and auditory clutter can be particularly limiting (Hiatt, 1982). A sensory cue which confuses or camouflages key objects can result in excessive confusion and/or catastrophic behavior (Yerxa and Baum, 1987). Even moderate degree of clutter in a household may present difficulty for the impaired person to identify salient cues. *The second basic intervention principle then is that the surroundings of a person with dementia need to be simple in order to offer accessible environmental information for orientation and navigation.*

C. Flexibility

The third dimension of objects, flexibility, is defined by Barris et al. as the "potential for using objects in a variety of ways" (Barris et al., 1985). Objects with flexibility can be used in different ways for several different tasks (e.g., consider the many roles of a knife on a camping trip). In dementia, flexibility can cause agitation, confusion or the misuse of objects. If an object appears applicable to several situations, cues about its intended use in any given context become blurred. *Thus, the third principle to guide intervention strategies is that expectations about object use should be static in order to afford the impaired person as much information as possible* (Breines, 1981).

D. Symbolic Meaning

The final dimension of the objects layer, symbolic meaning, refers to an object's representation of values, such as prestige, sex-role identification, age-appropriateness, and independence. There are many symbols of values in our society, and people with dementia may cherish these symbols more than previously, due to identity loss associated with disease. Objects required for a valued repetitive activity, such as whittling wood, carry many symbolic meanings. *A fourth intervention principle involves the understanding that the presence of age-appropriate materials and successful end products of a highly meaningful activity are important in maintaining ego integrity and as an outlet for expression of personal identity.*

TASK LAYER

The second environmental layer, tasks, refers to any sequence of action which satisfies either "external societal requirements or internal motives to explore and be competent" (Barris et al., 1985). Tasks include activities of work, self-care, or leisure, and tend to be goal-oriented and guided by rules for performance. The task layer has five dimensions which can be manipulated to influence arousal and press potentials of the individual and environment: complexity, temporal boundaries, rules, seriousness/playfulness, social implications.

A. Complexity

This dimension refers to skill level and the steps required for successful completion of a task. Individuals with moderate levels of dementia are often able to engage in a repetitive, gross-motor activity which requires no more than two to three steps for completion (Levy, 1987). Tasks can thus be simplified or graded down into components to facilitate completion by the impaired person. *The fifth basic principle is that task complexity can be mitigated by (1) emphasizing highly familiar, repetitive, gross-motor activities, and (2) using simplified, concrete verbal instructions which convey expected behavior. Augmenting instructions with non-verbal cues, demonstrating the desired action, or tactilely guiding an impaired person's hands can also facilitate communication* (Bartol, 1980; Berman and Rappaport, 1985; Levy, 1987).

B. Temporal Boundaries

Most individuals with dementia suffer from temporal disorientation and need assistance in the use of temporal cues from the environment (Oakley, 1987). Orienting cues from concrete representations of time or season must be highlighted to facilitate competence.

Dependable expectations about the order of the day are also critical so that one action gives rise to another. By establishing and following a dependable routine, multiple cues are gained from each event as to the sequence of necessary tasks (Levy, 1987). Hall and Buckwalter (1987) suggest individuals with dementia experience a progressively lowered stress threshold so that over the course of a day, stressful situations can accumulate to result in a catastrophic reaction. *A sixth basic principle involves providing special attention to a routine with frequent rest breaks in order to help reduce possibility of surpassing the stress threshold.* Furthermore, a weekly routine tends to establish a pattern which is comforting and informative to a person with dementia. Continued participation in routines, such as religious activities, structures time and conveys a sense of normalcy.

C. Rules

The third dimension, rules, is defined as the "internal organization of a task" (Barris et al., 1985) and refers to standards of performance. Rules may be clear and inflexible (as in a card game or sports activity) or vague and undefined (as in the role of a consultant). A person with dementia will often make mistakes but not recognize or correct errors. However, the emotional backlash from breaking a rule in a rigid environment is recognizable by an impaired adult. *A seventh principle for dementia is that criteria for success need to be clear and communicated to an impaired person in a variety of ways.* At the same time, rules should remain highly flexible to encourage exploration of surroundings for environmental cues about expected behavior. Caregivers can learn to identify rules in the household and eliminate or weaken those which negatively influence behavior of the impaired family member.

D. Seriousness/Playfulness

The fourth dimension relates to the seriousness or playfulness of the task and reflects societal expectations, the culture of family or immediate social group, and the context within which the task is performed. *In the case of cognitive impairment, the eighth intervention principle is that tasks must lack negative consequences and be non-anxiety provoking* (Levy, 1987; Oakley, 1987). Injecting playfulness to reduce tension is one technique for minimizing an anxiety producing task or the agitated behavior of the impaired person.

E. Social Dimension

The final dimension of the task layer concerns the public or private nature of activities and degree of competitiveness or cooperation involved. To sustain motivation to interact with the environment, tasks should be primarily cooperative, not competitive, and the outcome should benefit oneself or a highly approving other. Providing an impaired person with an atmosphere of unconditional positive regard can be a factor in reducing problem behaviors (Hall and Buckwalter, 1987).

Acceptable pastimes may involve time spent in passive activity, such as vicarious involvement in the events of the neighborhood by looking out the window. Time spent in this manner can assist the impaired person to remain part of the group (Sherman, LaGory and Ward, 1988). Rubinstein (1989) refers to the necessity of low-stimulus activity (daydreaming or "puttering") for defining and maintaining an individual's identity.

SOCIAL GROUPS AND ORGANIZATIONS

The third layer, social groups and organizations shapes the contents of the object and task layers, and in turn, these layers shape the characteristics of the social group. Four dimensions are critical to this layer: size, function, permeability, and structural complexity.

A. Size

Size of household membership tends to expand and shrink during the life cycle of a family and may have several implications for a caregiver and care recipient. There is no evidence to suggest that there is an optimal family size for functioning in the case of caring for an individual with dementia. However, size becomes critical in combination with other parameters, such as structural complexity. Birkel and Jones (1989) have concluded that the presence of several family members living in one residence tends to benefit the care recipient by providing more opportunities for productive activity engagement. The composition of the household is also important (non-family residents, frequent visitors, neighbors, etc.) and is addressed in the discussion of family function.

B. Function

The function of a family refers to the dominant occupation of the group, such as outside employment, child care or elder care. Developmental life tasks of the household effect behavioral expectations and actual performance of an impaired adult. For instance, several adults attempting to rise, eat, dress and leave by a certain time may lead to reluctance by an impaired person to acknowledge or act on his/her own needs.

There are usually critical shifts in responsibilities of family members as a consequence of the presence of dementia in the household. Not only are new work tasks created, but premorbid responsibilities of the individual with dementia must now be assumed by other family members. How a family solves the issue may depend upon resources, size, and the other dimensions of this layer.

C. Permeability

The function of a family is tied very closely to permeability or the extent to which a family incorporates formal supports (professional and other paid help) and informal supports (such as other family members, neighbors, and friends). Dementia strains the family's resources to the point that new resources may have to be cultivated in order to meet needs. Families will differ in their willingness to ask for and accept help from any outside source. *The ninth intervention principle speaks to the importance of determining how the needs of the family are being met, by whom, and how comfortable those involved are with the present arrangements.*

Soldo and Manton (1985) suggest two factors which predispose the use of formal supports by a caregiver: incontinence and need for specialized medical care. Their research indicates that use of the health care delivery system occurs only after the family's resources have been depleted. Hasselkus' (1987) research has also revealed that most caregivers use few if any formal supports due to a reluctance or unwillingness to share responsibility for care with a stranger (Hasselkus, 1987). In contrast, caregivers perceive engagement in a collaborative relationship with a health care professional to be a source of empowerment. In other words, through collaboration, caregivers become empowered or are enabled in their role as the primary care manager (Gitlin and Corcoran, in press). *The tenth intervention principle, therefore, is that the formal support worker must establish an atmosphere of collaboration by facilitating an open exchange of individual perspectives concerning problem identification and care strategies.*

D. Structural Complexity

The final dimension of the social group and organizations layer is structural complexity of the household. The structural complexity of the household may be very closely tied to other characteristics of the social group, such as permeability. It is important to assess how changes in one dimension will effect other dimensions, as well as determining total influence on other environmental layers.

A large household has the potential to allow variability in amount of time devoted to care provision, if approaches to care are coordinated. Conversely, a large disordered household with multiple caregivers may result in an inconsistent, disjointed and confusing care environment (Robinson, 1987). Each caregiver may have a different philosophy about care provision, preference for objects, and techniques for communicating instructions. Caregivers will also differ in the importance placed on assisting the care recipient in maintaining valued social contacts by invoking frequent visits by friends or non-resident family members (Zarit et al., 1980), especially since this adds to the structural complexity of the home. *The eleventh intervention principle involves identifying and training one family member to function as a care coordinator.* The care coordinator, with assistance of other formal and informal supports communicates decisions about care strategies to everyone involved in caring for the impaired individual. This coordinated approach to care is one necessary step toward shaping a consistent, competence-promoting environment for the family member with dementia.

CULTURE LAYER

The last environmental layer in Barris et al.'s model is familial culture. Cultural expectations about behavior which are internalized by the individual shape all choices about the contents and routines of daily life (Levine, 1987). As skills deteriorate, choices are limited and the impaired person confronts the loss of participation in meaningful life roles (Oakley, 1987). Yet, internalized expectations for behavior may not change and, in addition, caregiver expectations about his/her own and the spouse's behavior emerge as a very significant aspect of the environment. Relevant dimensions of the cultural layer include: nature of work and play, use of space and time, and transmission of knowledge and values.

A. Nature of Work and Play

Expectations about the value and acceptable forms of work and leisure, plus how much work and leisure are allowed to merge, create a range of possible influences (Barris et al., 1985). These expectations direct the efforts of the caregiver and care recipient to engage in valued activities. For most adults, a sense of productivity is highly valued and loss of productivity may create feelings of displacement.

B. Space/Time

Expectations about where and when activities should take place, issues of space and time, make up the second dimension of culture. Individuals usually influence to some degree space and activity timing, depending on their status in the household. Loss of that determination may signal a clear message about a new lowered status. What was formerly known as "Dad's chair" may be usable by anyone once Dad has dementia. In addition, people tend to order their homes in line with perceptions of sociocultural rules (Rubinstein, 1989), resulting in changes made in the home environment by the caregiver, based on his/her individual interpretation of being "sick" (Levine, 1987).

Related to space and time use expectations is value attached to non-productive time use. An individual's orientation toward time as circular, versus linear, may result in tolerance for rest periods or vicarious participation in the environment, such as watching activities of others through the window (Ward et al., 1988).

C. Transmission of Knowledge and Values

Finally, the third dimension of the cultural layer refers to transmission of knowledge and values. Important questions involve how a family defines the role of a person with dementia and how instructions for expected behavior in that role are communicated. A family may eliminate choice in the care recipient's life based on the belief that an individual with dementia is powerless and unable to exercise decisions.

Families tend to have a wide range of responses to dementia which may include fostering excessive levels of dependence, grieving and role transition. *The twelfth intervention principle which emerges from this dimension is the need to understand unique family processes and family caregiver styles as a critical aspect of the environment which effects caregiving and carerecipient behaviors.*

A CASE EXAMPLE

The following case material illustrates how environmental layers and respective dimensions exert interdependent influences upon the behavior of an impaired adult.

Background: Mrs. Y lives in a modest Northeast Philadelphia row home with her husband and five other adults. She is moderately to severely affected with Alzheimer's disease and is totally dependent in all self-care, work and leisure activities. She is unable to verbally communicate with others, and frequently cries in frustration. Mrs. Y's sociocultural atmosphere is very complex. Living in the home with Mr. and Mrs. Y are a quadriplegic son, a daughter, a boarder, and a son with a drug abuse problem. Although Mr. Y, who is retired, is the primary caregiver, everyone in the household is involved in caregiving to some degree (size and structural complexity).

Presenting Problem: The problem behavior addressed in Mrs. Y's case is urinary incontinence and the family reported she experienced in excess of 15 "accidents" per week. Usually before an accident occurred, Mrs. Y rose from where she was sitting and began to act very anxious. Within seconds, she was incontinent and often cried as she was led to the bathroom.

Influence of Object layer on problem behavior: The family's use of space and objects influences Mrs. Y's incontinence. In order to make room for a boarder, Mrs. Y was moved to a hospital bed in the living room (object symbolic meaning placed her in a "sick" role). The only bathroom was on the second floor (object availability), so a commode was obtained for Mrs. Y. Unfortunately, the commode was an unfamiliar object and because of her dementia, Mrs. Y was never able to associate it with her need to urinate (object complexity). The object's intended use became even more ob-

·scure when the family began placing a telephone on it for their easy access (object flexibility).

Influence of task and social groups layer: The tasks and activities of the family further influenced Mrs. Y's problem behavior in the area of toileting. The primary function of three of the members required them to leave the home early each morning. This created "peak" times for bathroom usage which others in the household tried to avoid (task temporal boundaries). Mrs. Y was sensitive to the impatience of others when she required the bathroom during these times (task rules). Although Mr. Y attempted to use humor to reduce Mrs. Y's anxiety about her needs (task seriousness/playfulness), other family members did not share his skill at this. For an impaired person in the Y's household, the task complexity of toileting was enormous.

Influence of sociocultural level: Unfortunately, the family members had not developed a consistent approach to Mrs. Y's incontinence, exposing her to a wide spectrum of caregiver knowledge, values, and care techniques (Mr. Y's approving attitude is contrasted with his son's impatience and misinformation).

Intervention Strategy: To address Mrs. Y's incontinence, basic environmental modifications were introduced and implemented. The identification of the problem and suggested modifications evolved from a collaborative process between an occupational therapist and Mr. Y over five home visits (Gitlin and Corcoran, in press; Corcoran, Schaumann, and Gitlin, 1990). First, Mr. Y began to articulate his caregiving style to the other family members to arrive at a more consistent approach to care of Mrs. Y (social groups layer). Household responsibilities were shifted so that only a few skillful family members were designated as Mrs. Y's caregivers (social groups layer). The occupational therapist and Mr. Y discovered that Mrs. Y was able to use her long-term memory to find the upstairs bathroom from her old bedroom, so plans were made to move her back upstairs (task layer). A bladder program was developed and implemented which avoided the "peak" bathroom times and thereby relaxed the rules associated with its usage (task layer). Mrs. Y was taken to the bathroom every 3 hours, instructions were conveyed tactilely and physical assistance was provided, reducing the task complexity of toileting. The family reduced the expectation that Mrs. Y could learn to use the commode and it was used only in emergency situations (object and social groups layers). The importance of simplifying the environment was conveyed to the family and the telephone was removed from the commode (object layer).

The outcome of this environmental approach was dramatic. Mrs. Y's accidents decreased from 15 to 3 incidents during the first week the changes were implemented. In a follow-up interview, the family reported the successful application of some of these same environmental principles to another self care problem, bathing.

CONCLUSIONS

This paper presents a model of the environment to understand transactions in households caring for an individual with dementia. The proposed model conceptualizes the environment as four concentric layers which form a hierarchy of influence on the behavior of the impaired person and their caregiver(s). The sociocultural atmosphere of the family will determine to a large extent the choice and presence of objects and tasks. The model generated twelve basic principles to guide development of specific interventions designed to optimize functioning of the impaired adult. These principles organize the wide range of care strategies which are available through manipulation of each dimension or combination of dimensions and layers. Directions for future research include examining the natural caregiving styles of individuals caring for a family member with dementia to determine the extent to which the full range of environmental adaptations are used. Additionally, rigorous testing of a skill building intervention for caregivers which instructs in the basic principles developed here is critical to establish the validity of the environmental model, and expand the range of services available to this population in need of support.

REFERENCES

Abels EK (1990). Informal care for the disabled elderly. *Research on Aging*, Newbury Park, CA.

Barris R, Kielhofner G, Levine R, and Neville A (1985). Occupation as interaction with the environment, in Kielhofner G, (ed). *A Model of Human Occupation: Theory and Application*, Williams and Wilkins, Baltimore.

Bartol MA, (1980). Nursing care of the patient with alzheimer's disease. Unpublished guidelines, Veterans Administration Medical Center, Tacoma, Washington.

Birkel RC, and Jones CJ (1989). A comparison of the caregiving networks of dependent elderly individuals who are lucid and those who are demented. *The Gerontologist*, Vol. 29(1), pp. 114-119.

Berman S, and Rappaport MB, (1984). Social work and alzheimer's disease: psychosocial management in the absence of a medical cure. *Social Work in Health Care*, Vol. 10(2), pp. 53-70.

Breines E (1981). *Perception: Its Development and Recapitulation*. Geri-Rehab, Lebanon, NJ.

Calkins MP, (1989). *Design for Dementia*. National Health Publishing, Owings Mills, MD.

Cohen GD and Crook T, (1989). Treating the older dementia patient. National Institute of Mental Health, Rockville, MD.

Corcoran MA, and Barrett, DA (1987). Using sensory integration principles with regressed elderly patients. *Sensory Integrative Approaches in Occupational Therapy*. The Haworth Press, Inc., New York.

Corcoran MA, Schaumann K, and Gitlin L (1990). Alzheimer's disease: a new service model to promote competent caregiver occupational behavior. Presentation at *Pennsylvania Occupational Therapy Annual Conference*, Philadelphia, PA.

Dawson P, Kline K, Wiancko DC, and Wells D (1986). Preventing excess disability in patients with alzheimer's disease. *Geriatric Nursing*, Nov./Dec., pp. 298-301.

Gallagher DE (1985). Intervention strategies to assist caregivers of frail elders: current research status and future research directions. *Annual Review of Gerontology and Geriatrics*, Vol. 5, 249-282.

Gitlin L, and Corcoran MA (in press). Focus on collaboration: training occupational therapists in the care of the elderly with dementia and their caregivers. *Educational Gerontology*, Washington, DC.

Hasselkus B (1988). Meaning in family caregiving: perspectives on caregiver/professional relationships. *The Gerontologist*, Vol. 28 (5).

Hiatt LG (1982). The environment as a participant in health care. *The Journal of Long-Term Care Administration*, Spring, pp. 1-17.

Hall GR, and Buckwalter, KC, (1987). Progressively lowered stress threshold: a conceptual model for care of adults with alzheimer's disease. *Archives of Psychiatric Nursing*, Vol. 1(6), pp. 399-406.

Institute of Medicine, (1988). *The Social and Built Environment in Older Society*, National Academy Press, Washington DC.

Lawton MP (1983). Environment and other determinants of well-being in older people. *The Gerontologist*, 23, pp. 349-357.

Lawton MP (1989). The impact of the environment on aging and behavior. In Birren and Schaie (eds), *Aging and Technology*, Plenum, Publishers, New York.

Lawton MP (1989). Environmental proactivity in older people. In Bengtson and

Schaie (eds), *The Course of Later Life: Research and Reflections*, Springer Publishers.

Lawton MP, and Nahemow LE, (1973). Ecology and the aging process. In Eisdorfer C, Lawton MP (eds), *The Psychology of Adult Development and Aging*. Washington DC, American Psychological Association.

Lawton MP, Brody EM, and Saperstein, AR (1989). A controlled study of respite service for caregivers of alzheimer's patients. *The Gerontologist*, Vol. 29, No. 1.

Levine RE (1987). Culture: a factor influencing the outcomes of occupational therapy. *Occupational Therapy in Health Care*, Spring, Vol. 4(1), pp. 3-16.

Levy LL, (1987). Psychosocial intervention and dementia: the cognitive disability perspective part 2. *Occupational Therapy in Mental Health*, Winter, Vol. 7(4), pp. 13-36.

Oakley, F (1987). Clinical application of the model of human occupation in dementia of the alzheimer's type. *Occupational Therapy in Mental Health*, Winter, Vol. 7(4), pp. 37-50.

Robinson, L (1987). Patient compliance in occupational therapy home health programs: sociocultural implications. *Occupational Therapy in Health Care*, Spring, Vol. 4(1), pp. 127-137.

Rogers JC, Marcus CL, and Snow TL (1987). Maude: a case of sensory deprivation. *American Journal of Occupational Therapy*, Vol. 41(10), pp. 673-676.

Rubinstein RL (1987). The significance of personal objects to older people. *Journal of Aging Studies*, Vol. 1(3), pp. 225-238.

Rubinstein RL, (1989). The home environments of older people: a description of the psychosocial processes linking person to place. *Journal of Gerontology: Social Sciences*, Vol. 44(2), pp. S45-53.

Select Committee on Aging, (1990). *Sharing the Caring: Options for the 90s and Beyond*. Committee Publishing No. 101-750, Washington DC.

Special Committee on Aging (1987). *Developments in Aging*, United States Senate Committee Publishing No. 0-291, Washington DC.

Soldo KG, and Manton BJ (1985). Dynamics of health changes in the oldest old: current patterns and future trends. *Milbank Memorial Fund Quarterly*, Spring, Vol. 63(2), pp. 286-319.

Stone R, Cafferata GL, and Sangl J, (1987). Caregivers of the frail elderly: a national profile. *The Gerontologist*, Vol. 27, No. 5.

Ward RA, LaGory M, Sherman SR (1988). *The Environment for Aging*. University of Alabama Press, Tuscaloosa, Alabama.

Yerxa EJ, and Baum S (1987). Environmental theories and the older person. *Topics in Geriatric Rehabilitation*, Vol. 3(1), pp. 7-18.

Zarit, SH, Reever, KE, and Bach-Peterson, J, (1980). Relatives of the impaired elderly: correlates of feelings of burden. *The Gerontologist*, Vol. 20(6), pp. 649-655.

Mental Health Issues in the Elderly

Victor A. Molinari, PhD

The elderly suffer from psychological difficulties at approximately the same rate as young adults. With the increasing number of those over the age of 65, combined with the 4% who have senile dementia (Mortimer, 1983), it is clear that elders and their families will be making expanding demands upon the mental health system (Blazer, 1989).

Professionals, elderly, and relatives of the elderly should be aware of the common psychological difficulties of the aged so that they can be rapidly and effectively assessed and treated. Unfortunately, psychiatric referrals are often not made until the problem has reached a crisis stage and hospitalization is inevitable. Preventative mental health care via outpatient visits to trained professionals aware of aging issues is a far too uncommon event. Older adults need to be educated that having an emotional problem is not synonymous with unalterable craziness and permanent institutionalization.

COMMON PSYCHOLOGICAL PROBLEMS

Depression

The most *common psychological problem* of the elderly is depression. Some researchers report that as many as 27% of elderly living in the community show some depressive symptoms, and 8% are significantly depressed (Blazer, Hughes, & George, 1987).

Victor A. Molinari is Staff Psychologist, Geropsychiatric Ward, Veterans Affairs Medical Center, Houston, TX.

23

Symptoms of depression include a sad mood, loss of appetite, poor sleeping (particularly early morning waking), guilt feelings, irritability, and suicidal thoughts. Elderly adults also present with concentration problems, preoccupation with physical symptoms, and memory complaints. The highest suicide rate of any age group is recorded for single white elderly males over the age of 60 (Katz, Curlik, & Nemetz, 1988) who have no social support system available to buffer the stresses of aging.

Hypochondriacal worries can be viewed as depression masked by physical complaints. Many older adults are ashamed to admit to emotional problems, so medical care allows them a socially acceptable access to nurturance from families and physicians. These "somaticizers" crave a great deal of attention from others, which need will eventually "turn off" those people who try to help them. Medical doctors will often enthusiastically accept such patients and perform a variety of different tests to evaluate their condition. When the results yield no identifiable pathology, the physicians feel they have wasted their time and reject them. The important point is that the elderly require regular attention and reassurance from mental health personnel to fill their interpersonal vacuum and reduce unnecessary medical intervention.

Depression must be differentiated from bereavement. For example, when a death occurs, it is natural to feel sad for a period of time. However, if mourning does not immediately occur, an individual may have a delayed grief reaction long after the loss has been suffered. This occurs particularly if an individual has been very dependent on the other and has had mixed feelings about the deceased person which prevents him/her from mourning the real relationship with its weaknesses as well as strengths.

Researchers have suggested that genetic vulnerability and changes in brain chemistry may play a role in severe depression, and psychological and social stressors interact with these biological variables in varying degrees to overwhelm the person. The most common precipitating events are losses that the elderly must confront: death of a spouse, close relatives, or friends; retirement; illness; parenting role; prestige; and independence. Those older adults who are quite dependent on others, or who are rigid and compulsive are more likely to become depressed in old age (Verwoerdt, 1981).

Some depressed people can become quite moody and swing from "lows" to "highs." Excess energy, talking too much or too rapidly, racing thoughts, grandiose ideas, spending too much money, and behaving with poor judgment are signs of mania which can occur, and should be treated, at any age (Molinari, Chacko, & Rosenberg, 1983).

Late Life Paranoid Disorders

Another major psychological problem amongst the elderly is *late life paranoid reactions* (Molinari & Chacko, 1983). Social isolation, subtle memory problems, and sensory defects can lead to increased suspiciousness and accusation of wrongdoing by others. Severe, full-blown psychotic delusions may develop along with auditory hallucinations. Unlike the depressive who berates himself for all his problems, the paranoid individual denies any responsibility for his difficulties and projects it onto others. Lifelong interpersonal oversensitivity may cause social isolation in old age which in turn leads to increasing misinterpretation of reality. These individuals rarely seek help for themselves and are often brought to mental health professionals by concerned relatives and/or by the legal system.

Alcoholism and Drug Abuse

Alcoholism in the elderly is probably less prevalent than in young adults (Myers et al., 1984), but will be a worse problem for those aged who do drink to excess because alcohol has longer lasting effects on the physical and mental status of the elderly. Two distinct groups of elderly alcoholics have been identified: early life or chronic alcoholics who have continued to drink as they have become older, and late life alcoholics who have begun drinking due to the losses sustained as they have aged. It has been proposed that the latter group has a better prognosis if their current social situation can be changed to help replace the losses (Dupree, Broskowski, & Schonfeld, 1984).

In addition to alcoholism, *prescription drug abuse* can cause excess disability in the elderly (Roberts, 1986). People over the age of 65 will often have at least one chronic condition which may require medication, and as age increases, more drugs are needed for an increasing number of physical ailments. Some older people may medicate themselves by buying over-the-counter drugs or changing the dosages of prescribed drugs without consulting their physician. Older adults with nervousness are often prescribed agents which are effective in dealing with the physiological effects of anxiety, but not in remediating the anxiety-provoking situation. Such drugs in high dosages taken over extended periods of time can be addictive and need to be monitored closely by physicians. Abuse of medication leading to dependence and/or confusion will often precipitate admission to a hospital for medication management.

Schizophrenia

Schizophrenia is *rarely first diagnosed* in late life, (Chistison, Chistison, & Blazer (1989), but many aged chronic schizophrenics are living in nursing homes because of the failure of the state hospital deinstitutionalization movement to provide adequate community care. Acute psychotic symptoms disrupt nursing home staff and residents and often precipitate psychiatric admissions. Professionals who work in nursing homes must be aware of the large number of residents with significant psychiatric problems so that their emotional needs can be as rapidly identified and treated as their physical needs.

DEMENTIA

Approximately half of the admissions to a geropsychiatric inpatient ward will be those diagnosed with *primary degenerative dementia* (PDD), i.e., a chronic usually irreversible gradual decline of general intellectual functioning, particularly memory, leading to changes in personality and behavior (Molinari, in press). The most common form of PDD is Alzheimer's Disease, where there is a deficiency in the brain chemical acetylcholine causing problems in the transfer of information from one brain cell to another (Coyle, 1985). A second type is multi-infarct dementia, or multiple small strokes in the brain caused by cerebrovascular disease. A third is communicative hydrocephalus where there is enlargement of the ventricles in the brain. Alcohol can also cause dementia. A thorough medical examination must be conducted to distinguish chronic dementia from acute confusion due to reversible physical causes and/or over-medication.

Dementia should also be distinguished from depression, which often has the same features of social withdrawal, moodiness, memory complaints, and loss of interest. For those suffering from depression, these signs stem from predominant negative emotions that are often associated with stressful precipitating events in the depressive's life, and are not due to the neurological deficits of Alzheimer's Disease. In general, depressed people emphasize memory difficulties while those with Alzheimer's Disease attempt to minimize them.

TREATMENT STRATEGIES

Treatment of the psychological difficulties of the elderly are as varied as the treatment for young adults. Each elder is an individual with his/her own strengths and weaknesses which should be thoroughly assessed so that a comprehensive treatment plan can be based on the aged person's unique circumstances. Therapy should be conceptualized from a biopsychosocial framework, with each component being addressed after a thorough evaluation of the medical, psychiatric, psychological, and social factors involved.

When psychological problems are so severe that they incapacitate the individual, biological treatments can be effective in getting the individual to think more clearly and to regulate moods. Antipsychotic medication for paranoid reactions, antidepressants for major depression, and lithium for bipolar disorder have been shown to be effective in treating these problems if used judiciously by psychiatrists trained in working with the elderly. The management of the interaction between psychotropic drugs and other medications for physical problems, and the evaluation of any medical causes of behavior change, are best conducted by coordination between the psychiatrist and other medical specialties.

Psychotherapy can be particularly effective in exploring the psychological problems of those elderly who are introspective, verbal, and motivated to change. Individual therapy will often focus on the stresses caused by the losses of aging. By allowing persons to freely express their emotions in a supportive atmosphere, the way can be paved for development of strategies to replace these losses. Stress management can teach elderly individuals better ways of thinking under pressure and more effective coping techniques to replace drug-taking behaviors.

Marital and/or family therapy may be necessary if the family situation is adding to the stress of adjustment to aging, rather than acting as an emotional buffer. Marital difficulties can occur when the husband retires and spends more time than ever at home with a wife unaccustomed to such closeness. New ways of interaction will need to be developed. Group therapy can provide a climate of emotional support and encouragement for change in those elderly experiencing common aging concerns. Life review reminiscence groups have been found to be helpful in sorting out the joys and sorrows of the past to aid the individual in embracing the future.

Social treatment can also be quite worthwhile in reducing the stressors causing psychological difficulties in the elderly. Financial, transportation, and social isolation problems can often be remedied by referral to social agencies for food stamps, Medicare or Medicaid assistance, transportation for the handicapped, and senior citizen centers.

PREVENTION

To *prevent* chronic psychological problems and psychiatric recidivism from occurring in the elderly, it is important to provide outreach programs to identify and evaluate those who have emotional problems before they become incapacitated, and to offer case management assistance to ensure continuity of care and enhance quality of life upon discharge. Since elders are often wary of mental health facilities, a trusted health worker can be invaluable in helping them negotiate the system so as to be comprehensively evaluated and regularly followed in order that they do not "fall between the cracks" and remain untreated.

Persons over the age of 65 comprise the most variable age group in a number of dimensions, particularly level of education, verbal skills, and socioeconomic status. On average, most older people are satisfied with their lives and concerned more with maintaining their quality of life than preoccupied with death and dying issues. The main goal of psychological treatment should always be to help elders regain some control and independence. There is no substitute for an accurate, detailed social/psychological/medical assessment to help determine which treatments in which combination can be most efficacious in helping the elderly live with dignity. Research has documented that psychotherapy with the aged is effective (Thompson, Gallagher, Steinmetz-Breckenridge 1987), and the earlier that problems are addressed the less likely that crises in care will occur.

REFERENCES

Blazer, D. (1989). The epidemiology of psychiatric disorders in late life. In E. Busse & D. Blazer (Eds.), *Geriatric psychiatry* (pp. 235-260). Washington, D. C.: American Psychiatric Press, Inc.

Blazer, D., Hughes, D. C., & George, L. K. (1987). The epidemiology of depression in an elderly community population. *The Gerontologist, 27,* 281-287.

Chistison, C., Chistison, G., & Blazer, D. (1989). Late life schizophrenia and paranoid disorders. In E. Busse & D. Blazer (Eds.), *Geriatric psychiatry* (pp. 403-414). Washington, D. C.: American Psychiatric Press, Inc.

Coyle, J. T. (1985). Cholinergic deficiencies in senile dementia of the Alzheimer type. In C. M. Gaitz & T. Samorajski (Eds.), *Aging 2000: Our health care destiny: Vol. 1. Biomedical issues* (pp. 213-219). New York: Springer-Verlag.

Dupree, L., Broskowski, H., & Schonfeld, L. (1984). The Gerontology alcohol project: A behavioral treatment program for elderly alcohol abusers. *The Gerontologist, 24* (5), 510-516.

Katz, I., Curlik, S., & Nemetz, P. (1988). Functional psychiatric disorders in the elderly. In L. Lazarus (Ed.), *Essentials of geriatric psychiatry: A guide for health professionals* (pp. 113-137). New York: Springer.

Molinari, V. (in press). Demographic and psychiatric characteristics of 390 consecutive discharges from a geropsychiatric inpatient ward. *Clinical Gerontologist.*

Molinari, V., & Chacko, R. (1983). The classification of paranoid disorders in the elderly: A clinical problem. *Clinical Gerontologist, 1* (4), 31-37.

Molinari, V., Chacko, R., Rosenberg, S. D. (1983). Bipolar disorder in the elderly. *Journal of Psychiatric Treatment and Evaluation, 5,* 325-330.

Mortimer, J. A. (1983). Alzheimer's disease and senile dementia: Prevalence and incidence. In B. Reisberg (Ed.), *Alzheimer's disease: The standard reference* (pp. 141-149). New York: Free Press.

Myers, J. K., Weissman, M. M., Tischler, G. L., Holzer, C. E., Leaf, P.J., Oruaschel, H., Anthony, J. C., Boyd, J. H., Burke, J.D., Kramer, M., &

Stoltzman, R. (1984). Six month prevalence of psychiatric disorders in three communities. *Archives of General Psychiatry, 41*, 959-969.

Roberts, A. H. (1986). Excess disability in the elderly: Exercise management. In L. Teri & P.M. Lewinsohn (Eds.), *Geropsychological assessment and treatment: Selected topics* (pp. 87-119). New York: Springer.

Thompson, L., Gallagher, D., & Steinmetz-Breckenridge, J. (1987). Comparative effectiveness of psychotherapies for depressed elders. *Journal of Consulting and Clinical Psychology, 55* (3), 385-390.

Verwoerdt, A. (1981). *Clinical geropsychiatry* (2nd ed.). Baltimore, MD.: The Williams-Wilkins Company.

Temporal Adaptation and Performance of Daily Living Activities in Persons with Alzheimer's Disease

Sheryl Denise Venable, MS, OTR/L
Marlys Marie Mitchell, PhD, OTR/L, FAOTA

SUMMARY. The purpose of this study was to investigate the relationships between temporal adaptation and functional capacity in persons with Alzheimer's Disease. The relationships were examined through the administration of research instruments designed to evaluate temporal orientation, organization and distortion, performance of activities of daily living (ADLs), and the severity of Alzheimer's Disease. The results demonstrated significant relationships between: (1) temporal adaptation and performance of ADLs: (2) temporal adaptation and severity of Alzheimer's Disease; and (3) the severity of Alzheimer's Disease and performance of ADLs. The findings suggested that as the Alzheimer's patient progresses through the course of the disease, temporal adaptation skills and performance of ADLs deteriorate progressively. The findings also suggested that temporal adaptation may predict ADL performance in persons with Alzheimer's Disease.

INTRODUCTION

Longevity is, for some, an exciting prospect. For others, it increases the fear of decline, gradual loss of function and, most distressing, loss of intellect. These people fear what society calls senility and dementia. Today medical science refers to the condition as Alzheimer's Disease. Alzheimer's Disease is a progressive, dementing disorder, usually of middle or late life, characterized by

---

Sheryl D. Venable is Occupational Therapist, North Carolina Baptist Hospital, Winston-Salem, NC.

Marlys M. Mitchell is Professor, Occupational Therapy Division, University of North Carolina, Chapel Hill, NC.

declining memory and other cognitive functions (McKhann, Drachman, Folstein, Katzman, Price and Stadlan, 1984). The loss of intellectual abilities and memory impairment may be severe enough to interfere with daily activities (APA, 1980).

For a diagnosis of Alzheimer's Disease, Roth (1982) believes three of the following four criteria must be satisfied: (1) Impairment in memory with difficulty in recording and retrieving recent personal experience and current information. (2) Deterioration in general intellectual ability with impairment of grasp, capacity for reasoning, inference and abstract thought. (3) Disorganization of personality with deterioration in self care, emotional blunting, disinhibition and a coarsening of behavior. (4) A gradual and progressive failure in the performance of work and in common activities of life, which is not attributable to other disease conditions.

The disease of the brain creates many problems in the Alzheimer's patient, including a loss of time perception (Mace and Rabins, 1981). Being unable to keep track of time, in turn, leads to problems in the organization of one's daily life (Kielhofner, 1977). There appears to be a relationship between time dysfunction and functional performance of daily living activities (ADL).

Assessment and intervention in ADLs is an area in which occupational therapy can make a contribution. Olin (1985) stated that the ability to perform self care activities is often the initial focus of evaluation with Alzheimer's patients. The person with Alzheimer's Disease will be able to care for himself in the early stages of the disease, but will gradually begin to neglect himself and eventually need help with bathing, dressing, grooming, feeding and oral hygiene (Mace and Rabins, 1981).

RELATING TEMPORAL ADAPTATION TO ADLs

Researchers (Mace and Rabins, 1981; Olin, 1985; Whitney, 1985) investigating Alzheimer's Disease have suggested several explanations for the breakdown in daily living activities in the Alzheimer's patient. However, an issue that has not been explored in the research is temporal adaptation. The purpose of this paper is to determine if temporal adaptation relates to the performance of daily living activities in the person with Alzheimer's Disease. Three specific research questions related to the purpose are:

1. Is there a significant correlation between temporal adaptation as measured by the Temporal Orientation Test, the Temporal Disorganization Scale and the Time Passage Test and the performance of daily living activities as measured by the Instrumental Activities of Daily Living – Physical Self Maintenance Scale?
2. Is there a significant correlation between temporal adaptation and the severity of Alzheimer's Disease as measured by the Hughes Evaluation Clinical Scale for Staging Dementia (CDR)?
3. Is there a significant correlation between the severity of Alzheimer's Disease and performance of daily living activities?

SUBJECTS

Procedures for Selection

The subjects involved in this study were identified through the Western North Carolina Chapter of the Alzheimer's Disease and Related Disorders Association (ADRDA), Mountain Geri-Care Center of Asheville, N.C., the Program on Aging in Chapel Hill and the Alzheimer's support groups of Chapel Hill and Asheville.

All the subjects were diagnosed by physicians as having Alzheimer's Disease. Subjects who met the following exclusionary criteria were not included in the study: (1) history of stroke or transient ischemic attack; (2) severe hypertension; (3) motor/neurologic disorder; (4) seizure disorder; (5) severe head trauma; (6) chronic/severe alcohol/drug abuse; (7) psychotic disorder; and (8) mental retardation.

Description of the Research Population

Descriptive data for the subjects participating in the study included sex, age, amount of education, living situation, residence, date of diagnosis and related medical conditions.

Out of 174 pairs of potential subjects and caregivers, contacted by telephone, nineteen subjects and their caregivers participated in both testing sessions; the remaining caregivers/subjects would not volunteer for the study. The subjects ranged in age from 50 to 97 years old with a diagnosis of Alzheimer's Disease dating from 1983 to August, 1987. Four subjects lived in nursing homes while the remaining fifteen subjects lived at home. Most of the subjects, 78.9 percent, were married, and 73.6 percent were living with a spouse or child.

INSTRUMENTATION

The Hughes Evaluation Clinical Scale
for Staging Dementia (CDR)

The Hughes CDR (Hughes et al., 1982), provides an in-depth and complete picture of the patient with Alzheimer's Disease through a global rating of abstract abilities, personal care, community affairs, home life and performance on task. This rating defines the patient's level/severity of dementia.

Inter-rater reliability for the CDR was found to be .89. The CDR showed strong correlations with previously devised dementia ratings (Dementia scale = .74, Face-Hand Test = .57 and the SPMSQ = .84). Validity, in contrast, was difficult to test due to the lack of assessments available that rate dementia.

Scoring the Hughes CDR involved assigning subjects a rating of: healthy (CDRO), mild (CDR1), moderate (CDR2), or severe dementia (CDR3). A rating of questionable dementia (CDR0.5) was included for subjects who were neither clearly demented nor healthy. All the information from the interviews and observations were used to score each category (M = Memory; O = Orientation; JPS = Judgement and Problem Solving; CA = Community Affairs; HF = Home Functions; PC = Personal Care), as independently as possible.

The Temporal Orientation Test (TOT)

The Temporal Orientation Test (Benton, VanAllen and Fogel, 1964), is a sensitive indicator of the presence of temporal disorientation. Reliability and validity data on the TOT are not available.

The score from the TOT was obtained by subtracting points from a perfect score of 100 (i.e., one point subtracted for each day away from the correct day). Temporal orientation scores of 97-100 were considered normal, 96-95 were considered moderately defective, and 94 or less grossly defective.

The Temporal Disorganization Scale (TDS)

The Temporal Disorganization Scale (Melges and Freeman, 1977), reflects alterations in the rate, sequential-ordering and goal-directedness of thinking processes in individuals. Reliability and validity data on the TDS are not available.

Subjects replied to the 20 statements on the TDS in terms of their experiences on the day of testing on the following scale: $0 =$ none, $1 =$ occasionally (1-2 times per hour), $2 =$ often (5-10 times per hour), $3 =$ frequently (more than 20 times per hour). A total score of temporal disorganization (ranging from 0 to 60) was then obtained by adding the individual scores. The higher the score, the more temporal disorganization was present.

The Test of Time Passage (TPT)

The Test of Time Passage (Coheen, 1950), measures the subject's ability to estimate the passage of short periods of time. Reliability and validity data on the TPT are not available.

In the TPT, each subject's estimates of time passage were compared to the established norms. The subject's ability to measure the passage of time was identified as: normal, pathologic underestimation, pathologic overestimation, or a loss of continuity. For the purposes of data analysis the number 0 was assigned to the "normal" category, 1 to "pathologic underestimation," 2 to "pathologic overestimation" and 3 to "loss of temporal continuity."

The Instrumental Activities of Daily Living Physical Self Maintenance Scale (IADL-PSMS)

The IADL-PSMS (Lawton and Brody, 1969), evaluates the functional abilities of elderly persons on different levels of competence, in particular, physical and instrumental autonomy in activities of daily living.

In the IADL-PSMS, the scores for both scales were determined by information obtained from the primary caregiver. The scoring systems used by Lawton and Brody (1969) have been altered by Heying (1983). The score for each item, which represents the level of specific activity competence attained, was computed. On the IADL, the total score, ranging from 0 to 23, was obtained by totaling subscores (0 = dependent through 4 = independent) from each test item. On the PSMS, the total score, ranging from 0 to 24, was obtained by totaling item subscores. The higher the score, the more independent the subject is in performing ADLs. These scores could be combined for a possible total score of 47. Norms and reliability data for the IADL-PSMS are unavailable using the revised scoring criteria by Heying (1983).

The validity of the IADL-PSMS is supported by significant correlations (.01 level) between the IADL and PSMS and three other functional measures: Physical Classification, Mental Status Questionnaire, and Behavior and Adjustment Rating Scales.

In spite of some limitations in availability of reliability and validity data, the instruments measuring temporal adaptation (Temporal Orientation Test, Temporal Disorganization Scale, and Time Passage Test), represent the few measurement sources available. They were selected because they are relevant to the sample being studied and because they may contribute important information on the temporal characteristics of persons with Alzheimer's Disease.

TEST ADMINISTRATION AND PROCEDURE

Each subject's caregiver was contacted by telephone and informed of the purpose of the study and the testing procedure and that the testing required two separate sessions.

In the first session, immediately preceding the testing, descriptive data on the subject was obtained from medical charts and/or the subjects' caregivers. Subjects and their primary caregivers were asked to sign informed consent forms. Each subject completed the temporal adaptation tests. The order in which the tests were administered was predetermined by using a random numbers chart in order to avoid a sequencing effect. The standardized test directions were read aloud immediately preceding each test. The subject's primary caregiver was asked to complete the IADL-PSMS to rate the subject's functional abilities in self care and instrumental activities of daily living.

A second session was conducted within the next seven days to administer the Hughes CDR.

Actual time spent with each subject and caregiver averaged 40 minutes for the first testing session and 90 minutes for the second session.

DATA ANALYSIS

Data were analyzed using the Spearman rank-order correlation coefficient and descriptive statistics. The Spearman correlation test used the medians of the test scores as the population statistic, since the data were converted to ranks. The established level of significance was $p < .05$.

RESULTS

Each subject's performance on the Hughes CDR, the TOT, the TDS, the TPT and the caregiver's ratings on the IADL-PSMS was tabulated (Table 1).

Question I: Is there a significant correlation between temporal adaptation and performance of daily living activities? The subjects' performance on the TOT were significantly related to the IADL scores of the IADL-PSMS (Table 2).

The subjects' performance on the TDS were significantly related to the PSMS scores of the IADL-PSMS and the total IADL-PSMS scores (Table 3).

The subjects' performance on the TPT was significantly related

TABLE 1

Individual Test Scores for Subjects with Alzheimer's Disease
(n=19)

Subj.	Hughes CDR	TOT	TDS	TPT	IADL	PSMS	IADL-PSMS
1	0.5	100	1	0	10	24	34
2	1	97	34	2	5	12	17
3	2	96	29	3	2	11	13
4	1	95	12	0	4	21	25
5	1	100	19	0	5	13	18
6	2	89	26	2	2	9	11
7	2	49	-3	0	2	19	21
8	1	92	1	0	3	18	21
9	0.5	98	15	2	19	22	41
10	0.5	99	10	0	4	22	26
11	2	45	25	3	1	15	16
12	2	33	2	2	4	15	19
13	2	75	23	2	0	13	13
14	1	45	16	2	16	23	39
15	2	89	17	2	1	14	15
16	0.5	95	7	0	14	23	37
17	2	85	23	2	2	11	13
18	1	95	17	0	5	18	23
19	1	97	12	0	7	18	25

to the PSMS scores of the IADL-PSMS and to the total IADL-PSMS scores (Table 4).

Question II: Is there a significant correlation between temporal adaptation and the severity of Alzheimer's Disease? The subject's scores on the TOT and the TPT were significantly related to the scores on the Hughes CDR (Table 5).

Question III: Is there a significant correlation between the severity of Alzheimer's Disease and performance of daily living activities? The subjects' scores on the Hughes CDR were significantly
related to the IADL scores of the IADL-PSMS, the PSMS scores of

Table 2

Rank Correlations Between the Temporal Orientation Test and the
Instrumental Activities of Daily Living-Physical Self
Maintenance Scale (n=19)

Rank correlation coefficient	TOT & IADL	TOT & PSMS	TOT& IADL-PSMS
Spearman	.499*	.193	.336
p values	.0295	.428	.160

*significant at .05 level

Table 3

Rank Correlations Between the Temporal Disorganization Test and
the Instrumental Activities of Daily Living-Physical Self
Maintenance Scale (n=19)

Rank correlation coefficient	TDS & IADL	TDS & PSMS	TDS & IADL-PSMS
Spearman	-.337	-.75*	-.65*
p values	.1586	.0002	.0023

*significant at .05 level

the IADL-PSMS, and to the total IADL-PSMS scores (Table 6).

To summarize, the data indicate significant correlations between the Temporal Orientation Test and the Instrumental Activities of Daily Living section of the Instrumental Activities of Daily Living-Physical Self Maintenance Scale; the Temporal Disorganization Scale and the PSMS section and the total IADL-PSMS; the TOT and the Hughes Clinical Dementia Rating; the Time Passage Test and the Hughes CDR; the Hughes CDR and the IADL and PSMS sections and the total IADL-PSMS. These results are summarized in Figure 1.

The subjects' performance of daily living activities are examined more closely in Tables 7 and 8. The percentages of subjects who completed the ADLs independently or with minor assistance are identified (Table 7). Physical self maintenance activities of feeding, toileting and ambulation were the least difficult activities for the Alzheimer's subjects. Percentages of subjects who performed the ADLs dependently or with major assistance are identified (Table 8). Activities of transportation, handling finances, food preparation and laundering were the most difficult for the total subject sample.

The subjects are grouped according to their Alzheimer's Disease severity level (Hughes CDR) and their test results are averaged

Table 4

Rank Correlations between the Time Passage Test and the Instrumental Activities of Daily Living-Physical Self Maintenance Scale (n=19)

Rank correlation coefficient	TPT & IADL	TPT & PSMS	TPT & IADL-PSMS
Spearman	-.41	-.542*	-.536*
p values	.083	.016	.018

*significant at .05 level

within each Hughes CDR category (Table 9). From Table 1, the subjects' Hughes CDR scores and individual test scores were used to group the subjects according to the Hughes CDR ratings and to average the test results within each Hughes CDR category in Table 9. Table 9 shows the average test scores for subjects classified by

Table 5

Rank Correlations Between the Temporal Orientation Test, the Temporal Disorganization Scale, the Time Passage Test and the Hughes Evaluation Clinical Scale for Staging Dementia (n=19)

Rank correlation coefficient	TOT & Hughes CDR	TDS & Hughes CDR	TPT & Hughes CDR
Spearman	-.71*	.41	.59*
p values	.0007	.077	.0077

*significant at .05 level

Table 6

Rank Correlations Between the Hughes Evaluation Clinical Scale for Staging Dementia and the Instrumental Activities of Daily Living-Physical Self Maintenance Scale (n=19)

Rank correlation coefficient	Hughes CDR IADL	Hughes CDR PSMS	Hughes CDR IADL-PSMS
Spearman	-.83*	-.73*	-.84*
p values	.0001	.0004	.0001

*significant at .05 level

the Hughes CDR ratings of questionable, mild, or moderate dementia. There were considerable differences in the average test scores between the different CDR categories. This table illustrates that as the subject's dementia increases, his performance on the tests deteriorates.

DISCUSSION

Subject Participation

Each subject completed all of the tests in this study. Although motor and neurological impairments were ruled out by the selection criteria, three subjects manifested visual impairments and two subjects had auditory difficulties.

Six of the nineteen subjects were tested alone at the request of the caregivers, while the remaining thirteen subjects were tested in the

---

Significant Correlations Exist Between:

TEMPORAL ADAPTATION AND PERFORMANCE OF ADL'S

(+) 1. Temporal Orientation Test and IADL

(-) 2. Temporal Disorganization Scale and PSMS

(-) 3. Temporal Disorganization Scale and IADL-PSMS

(-) 4. Time Passage Test and PSMS

(-) 5. Time Passage Test and IADL-PSMS

TEMPORAL ADAPTATION AND SEVERITY OF ALZHEIMER'S DISEASE

(-) 1. Temporal Orientation and Hughes CDR

(+) 2. Time Passage Test and Hughes CDR

SEVERITY OF ALZHEIMER'S DISEASE AND PERFORMANCE OF ADL'S

(-) 1. Hughes CDR and IADL

(-) 2. Hughes CDR and PSMS

(-) 3. Hughes CDR and IADL-PSMS

Figure 1. Summary of significant correlations

caregivers' presence. The caregivers of the six subjects tested alone expressed the subjects' tendencies to rely on the caregivers to answer questions asked of the subjects. The caregivers did not respond to the questions.

Instrumentation

Each subject was able to complete the TOT, the TDS, the TPT and the Hughes CDR. The tests were appropriate for the Alzheimer's subject sample, with the possible exception of the TDS due to the subjects' difficulties understanding directions and questions and determining valid answers. The IADL-PSMS seemed to be an appropriate scale for caregivers to rate the Alzheimer's subjects' abilities to perform daily living activities.

Temporal Adaptation and Performance of ADLs

The results of the tests indicated that there was a significant positive correlation between the TOT and the IADL section of the IADL-PSMS at the .05 level. The statistical comparisons also showed significant negative correlations at the .05 level between the TDS and the PSMS section of the IADL-PSMS and the total IADL-PSMS. The test results indicated significant negative correlations between the TPT and the PSMS and the total IADL-PSMS at the .05 level. "Normal" or "healthy" performances on the tests were represented by high scores on the TOT and the IADL-PSMS, and low scores on the TDS and TPT.

The lack of significant correlations between the TOT and the PSMS section of the IADL-PSMS and the total IADL-PSMS suggests that a meaningful relationship does not exist between temporal orientation and performance of self care activities in this sample of Alzheimer's subjects. This finding is contrary to the writings of Mace and Rabins, (1981) and Whitney (1985) who discuss the Alzheimer's patient's breakdown in temporal orientation and the effect it has on the patient's ability to dress appropriately and bathe, groom, toilet and feed regularly.

The significant negative correlation between the TDS and the PSMS section of the IADL-PSMS suggests a relationship between temporal organization and performance of self care activities in this

Table 7

Percentages of Subjects Who Performed IADL and PSM Activities
Independently or with Minor Assistance (n=19)

Activity	Independence or minor assistance in activity (% of subjects)
IADL Ability to use telephone	31.58
Shopping	10.53
Food preparation	10.53
Housekeeping	15.79
Laundry	10.53
Mode of transportation	5.26
Responsibility for own medication	15.79
Ability to handle finances	5.26
PSMS Toilet	84.21
Feeding	89.47
Dressing	42.11
Grooming	36.84
Physical ambulation	63.16
Bathing	52.63

sample. As the Alzheimer's patient loses his ability to sequence and organize his thoughts and actions in time, he may begin experiencing difficulty in performing his self care activities independently. These results are similar to assumptions made by Mace and Rabins (1981) and Whitney (1985), that expressed the impact of temporal disorganization on performance of self care activities in Alzheimer's patients.

Table 8

Percentages of Subjects Who Performed IADL-PSM Activities
Dependently or with Major Assistance (n=19)

Activity	Dependence or major assistance in activity (% of subjects)
IADL Ability to use telephone	21.05
Shopping	36.84
Food preparation	78.95
Housekeeping	73.68
Laundry	78.95
Mode of transportation	94.74
Responsibility for own medication	73.68
Ability to handle finances	89.47
PSMS Toilet	5.26
Feeding	0.00
Dressing	42.11
Grooming	36.84
Physical ambulation	10.53
Bathing	26.32

The nonsignificant correlation between the TDS and the IADL scale may be explained by two factors: the subjects' living situation and the caregivers' ratings of the subjects on the IADL-PSMS. The living situation for the majority of the subjects includes living at home. Their abilities to perform regular household activities such as housekeeping, laundering and food preparation, may be better than expected due to the familiarity of their home environment.

Table 9

Mean Test Scores for Subjects Classified by Hughes CDR

CDR	TOT	TDS	TPT	IADL	PSMS	IADL-PSMS
0.5*	98	8.25	0.50	11.75	22.75	34.5
1.0^	88.71	15.86	0.57	6.43	17.57	24.0
2.0^	70.12	17.75	2.0	1.75	13.5	15.25

*0.5 = questionable dementia (n=4)

^1.0 = mild dementia (n=7)

^2.0 = moderate dementia (n=8)

The second factor is the caregivers' ratings of the subjects on the IADL-PSMS. Biased scoring may have influenced the scores on the IADL-PSMS. The caregivers may have attempted to portray the subjects as healthier people than they actually were or they may have been uncertain of the subjects' performance levels in particular activities (such as laundering, housekeeping and food preparation), and may have rated them more independent than they actually were.

The significant negative correlation between the TPT and the PSMS implies that as the Alzheimer's patient becomes unable to measure the passage of time, he may fail to perform his self care activities regularly. This finding supports Mace and Rabins' (1981) hypothesis that being able to measure time passage influences the ability to feed, bathe, toilet, groom and change clothes regularly.

To summarize, these significant correlations suggest the Alzheimer's patient's abilities to know the day, month, date of month, year and time of day, to order and execute thoughts and actions in time, and to measure time passage may influence his ability to perform self care and independent living activities.

TEMPORAL ADAPTATION AND SEVERITY
OF ALZHEIMER'S DISEASE

The test results indicated a significant negative correlation between the TOT and the Hughes CDR at the .05 level. This implies that subjects who tested as being temporally oriented tested as having less severe dementia or, subjects who tested as being temporally disoriented tested as having more severe dementia. Alzheimer's patients early in the disease process begin to lose the ability to know the day, month, date of month, year and time of day. This ability progressively worsens as the disease progresses. This finding supports writings of Hughes et al. (1982); Mace and Rabins (1981); Reisberg, Ferris and Anand (1984); Whitney (1985); Winograd and Jarvik (1986); and Winogrond and Fisk (1983). These authors have found increased temporal disorientation in Alzheimer's patients as the patients progress through the disease stages. The relatively strong significant correlation between the TOT and the Hughes CDR may have resulted because both tests examine the subject's orientation in time. The TOT contains similar orientation questions as those stated in the Hughes CDR, thus making a correlation more likely.

There was also a significant positive correlation at the .05 level between the TPT and the Hughes CDR. This signifies that subjects who had the ability to measure time passage also tested as having less severe dementia. The Alzheimer's patient's decreased ability to measure the passage of time as their illness progresses seems logical and expected.

The lack of significant correlation between the TDS and the Hughes CDR is contrary to the writings of Cummings and Benson (1986); Mace and Rabins (1981); Rosen, Mohs and Davis (1984); Whitney (1985); and Winograd and Jarvik (1986). The lack of correlation between the TDS and the Hughes CDR may be due to the difficulties this sample of Alzheimer's subjects encountered with the TDS. The subjects' difficulties in understanding the test directions and questions and determining valid answers may have generated results not representative of the subject's temporal organization skills.

SEVERITY OF ALZHEIMER'S DISEASE
AND PERFORMANCE OF ADLs

The significant negative correlations between the Hughes CDR and the IADL scale, the Hughes CDR and the PSMS, and the Hughes CDR and the total IADL-PSMS imply that subjects who tested as having less severe dementia also performed ADLs independently/with minor assistance or, subjects who tested as having more severe dementia also performed ADLs dependently/with major assistance. It also suggests a relationship between the severity of Alzheimer's Disease and performance of ADLs. These findings are similar to the findings of Heying (1985); Hughes et al. (1982); Mace and Rabins (1981); Olin (1985); Reisberg, Ferris and Franssen (1985); Whitney (1985); and Winogrond and Fisk (1983). Both the Hughes CDR and the IADL-PSMS rely on the ratings of the caregiver, who directly observe the subject perform daily living activities in their natural environment. With both tests measuring the Alzheimer's subjects' performance of daily living activities, and both measurements obtained from the caregiver, the significant correlations between the Hughes CDR and the IADL-PSMS are more likely to occur.

Findings Associated with Individual
Items on the IADL-PSMS

The Alzheimer's subjects participating in this study demonstrated greater losses in the performance of instrumental activities of daily living (telephone usage, shopping, food preparation, housekeeping, laundry, transportation, handling medication and finances) than in the performance of physical self maintenance activities (toileting, feeding, dressing, grooming, ambulation and bathing). The average IADL score for the subject sample was 5.58, 24% of the maximum score of 23. The average PSMS score was 16.89, 70% of the maximum score of 24 (Table 7). Competence in these routine tasks have been developed since early childhood. It is likely that these tasks are retained the longest in subjects with Alzheimer's disease, because of their familiarity, their habitual performance over many years, and because the caregiver may tend to encourage the subject's participation in these basic activities that sustain life, a sense of privacy and dignity.

Independent living activities of transportation, handling finances, laundering, food preparation, housekeeping and handling medication ranked the highest in dependent performance by the subject sample (Table 8). It is probable that these activities are not retained because of their cognitive requirements, their decreased familiarity and because of safety concerns—cautious caregivers may perform these activities in order to avoid potential dangerous accidents. These results are similar to those of Heying's (1985) who reported greater loss in performance of IADLs than in self care activities in subjects with senile dementia.

When the subjects were grouped according to their Hughes CDR scores, and individual test scores (Table 1) were compared to the averages for each Hughes CDR category (Table 9), several subjects had scores notably higher or lower than other subjects in the same Hughes CDR category. These subjects' scores demonstrate the variable course that is characteristic of Alzheimer's Disease. Writings by Blass et al. (1983) and Carnes (1985) discuss the unpredictability of Alzheimer's symptoms and state that no two Alzheimer's patients experience the same progressive deteriorations in the course of the disease. A patient classified at a specific stage of Alzheimer's disease may exhibit symptomatic differences from others also at that stage. The variability described may be critical to understanding the group data presented in this study, as such data masks individual differences. Despite the temporal adaptation and IADL-PSMS score variations among the subjects in each Hughes CDR category, relationships exist between: temporal adaptation and the severity of Alzheimer's Disease; and performance of ADLs and the severity of the disease.

SUMMARY AND CONCLUSIONS

The results of this study demonstrated relationships between: (1) temporal adaptation and performance of daily living activities; (2) temporal adaptation and the severity of Alzheimer's Disease; and (3) the severity of Alzheimer's Disease and performance of daily living activities.

The information generated by this study regarding the temporal adaptation skills that influence performance of daily living activities in the Alzheimer's patient suggests the importance of further research in these areas. The results of this study, coupled with the results of future research, may lead to greater knowledge of the impact temporal dysfunction has on the Alzheimer's patient's functional capacities. Also, the findings from this study and future research may lead to the utilization of temporal adaptation tests and ADL scales as integral parts of the assessment and treatment of persons with Alzheimer's Disease. These types of assessments could be important to families and health professionals, for it is generally inability to perform daily living activities that is important in determining whether an individual requires institutionalization.

REFERENCES

American Psychiatric Association: *Diagnostic and Statistical Manual of Mental Disorders. 3rd Ed.* (DSM-III), Washington, D.C. Task Force on Nomenclature and Statistics, American Psychiatric Association, 1980.

Benton, A., VanAllen, M., and Fogel, M. (1964). Temporal orientation in cerebral disease; *Journal of Nervous and Mental Disorders, 139,* 110-119.

Blass, J., Cohen, G., Drachman, D., Folstein, M., and Katzman, R. (1983). Alzheimer's disease — the human dimension. In R. Katzman (Ed.), *Banbury Report, Biological Aspects of Alzheimer's Disease* (pp. 7-28). Cold Spring Harbor Laboratory.

Carnes, M. (1984). Diagnosis and management of dementia in the elderly. *Physical and Occupational Therapy in Geriatrics, 3,* 11-23.

Coheen, J., (1950). Disturbances in time discrimination in organic brain disease. *Journal of Nervous and Mental Disorders, 112,* 121-129.

Cummings, J., and Benson, D. (1986). Dementia of the Alzheimer's type: an inventory of diagnostic clinical features. *Journal of the American Geriatrics Society, 34,* 12-19.

Heying, L. (1985). Research with subjects having senile dementia. In C. Allen (Ed.) *Occupational Therapy for Psychiatric Diseases: Measurement and Management of Cognitive Disabilities* (pp. 339-365). Boston: Little, Brown and Company.

Hughes, S., Berg, L., Danzinger, W., Coben, L, and Martin, R. (1982). A new clinical scale for the staging of dementia. *British Journal of Psychiatry, 140,* 556-572.

Kielhofner, G. (1977). Temporal adaptation: a conceptual framework for occupational therapy. *American Journal of Occupational Therapy, 31,* 235-242.

Lawton, M., and Brody, E. (1969). Assessment of older people: self-maintaining and instrumental activities of daily living. *Gerontologist, 9,* 179-186.

McKhann, G., Drachman, D., Folstein, M., Katzman, R., Price, D., Stadlan, E. (1984). Clinical Diagnosis of Alzheimer's Disease: Report of the NINCDS-ARDA Work Group under the auspices of Department of Health and Human Services Task Force on Alzheimer's Disease. *Neurology, 34,* 939-944.

Mace, N., and Rabins, P. (1981). *The 36-Hour Day.* Baltimore: Johns Hopkins Press.

Melges, F., and Freeman, A. (1977). Temporal disorganization and inner-outer confusion in acute mental illness. *American Journal of Psychiatry, 30,* 874-877.

Olin, D. (1985). Assessing and assisting the persons with dementia: an occupational behavior perspective. *Physical and Occupational Therapy in Geriatrics, 3,* 25-32.

Reisberg B., Ferris, S., and Anand, R. (1984). Functional staging of dementia of the Alzheimer's type. *Annals of the New York Academy of Science, 435,* 481-483.

Reisberg B., Ferris, S., and Franssen, E. (1985). An ordinal functional assessment tool for Alzheimer's-type dementia. *Hospital and Community Psychiatry, 36,* 593-595.

Rosen, W., Mohs, R., and Davis, K. (1984). A new rating scale for Alzheimer's disease. *American Journal of Psychiatry, 141,* 1356-1364.

Roth, M. (1982). Perspectives in the diagnosis of senile and pre-senile dementia of the alzheimer type. In M. Sarner (Ed.) *Advanced Medicine, Vol. 18.* London: The Royal College of Physicians and Pitman Medical.

Whitney, F. (1985). Alzheimer's disease: toward understanding and management. *Nurse Practitioner, 10,* 15-36.

Winograd, C., and Jarvik, L. (1986). Physician Management of the Demented Patient. *Journal of the American Geriatric Society, 34,* 295-308.

Winogrond, I., and Fisk, A. (1983). Alzheimer's disease: Assessment of functional status. *Journal of the American Geriatrics Society, 31,* 780-785.

Constructional Apraxia
in Alzheimer's Disease:
Contributions to Functional Loss

Dorothy F. Edwards, PhD
Carolyn M. Baum, MA, OTR
Ruthmary K. Deuel, MD

INTRODUCTION

Functional loss and complete dependence are commonly accepted as the inevitable consequences of senile dementia of the Alzheimer type (SDAT). Although the loss of functional ability is present even at the mild stage of the disease, the factors associated with functional disability in this population are not well understood. While memory impairment is the primary feature of Alzheimer's disease, many other cognitive skills are affected, and each of these effects contributes in some way to the progressive loss of functional competence. Little is known about the differential impact of factors such as apraxia on the performance of daily life tasks in this population.

The purpose of this paper is to explore the relationship of con-

Dorothy F. Edwards and Carolyn M. Baum are affiliated with the Alzheimer's Disease Research Center, the Program in Occupational Therapy and the Department of Neurology, Washington University School of Medicine, St. Louis, MO 63110. Ruthmary K. Deuel is affiliated with the Alzheimer's Disease Research Center, the Department of Neurology and the Department of Pediatrics, Washington University School of Medicine, St. Louis, MO 63110.

Address correspondence to Dorothy F. Edwards, Program in Occupational Therapy, Box 8066, 4567 Scott Ave., St. Louis, MO 63110.

This research was supported in part by the National Institute on Aging, Grant # AGO3391.

53

structional apraxia to ADL performance across the stages of Alzheimer's disease. It is hoped that a better understanding of this relationship will help therapists working with SDAT patients and their families.

REVIEW OF THE LITERATURE

In its simplest form, constructional apraxia is defined as difficulty in assembling one-dimensional units into two-dimensional figures or patterns. While this type of deficit has been widely recognized and described in clinical populations, the nature of constructional apraxia and the types of assessment techniques used with patients have both raised considerable speculation and debate.

Constructional apraxia was not considered a separate disorder with a distinct neuropsychological significance until 1934. Kleist (1934) viewed constructional apraxia as an inability to translate visual perceptions into appropriate motor activity, such that the spatial part of the task was missed. Similarly, van der Horst (1934) emphasized the execution of an act, suggesting that constructional apraxia appeared when there was an interference with an action, especially with action such as putting together a puzzle, copying a drawing, or building with bricks. Critchley (1971) in his review of constructional apraxia concluded that clinically it lies outside the category of most other varieties of apraxia, and that constructional apraxia is an executional deficit within the visuospatial domain.

Theoretically, it is hypothesized that constructional apraxia results from damage to the brain's linkage between the visual image of an object and the mental image of a movement using that object. Constructional apraxia differs from other forms of visual disorientation in that the patient is unable to perform a motor task correctly within a visual sphere. Many patients appear not to have other forms of visual spatial dysfunction (Critchley, 1971). Mayer Gross (1935) hypothesized that constructional apraxia represented a particular expression of space impairment, involving "activity space" within the sphere of hand and fingers. Thus, constructional apraxia involves elements of both apraxic or executional skills and gnostic or perceptual function.

Measurement of Constructional Praxis

The measurement of constructional apraxia has not been standardized. Usually constructional apraxia is assessed by two dimensional tasks (e.g., design copying, drawing simple geometric shapes and block designs such as the Kohs designs). The difficulty of such tasks varies and the performance of patients differs widely. Many patients displaying constructional deficits do reasonably well on simple tasks such as drawing geometric figures but fail more complex tasks such as block construction (Benton, 1967). Also, patient performances vary between the ability to spontaneously execute a drawing at the suggestion of an examiner and the patient's ability to copy a drawing (Critchley, 1971).

Most studies of constructional apraxia have relied solely on two-dimensional tasks. The importance of moving from two-dimensional to three-dimensional tasks was first raised by Critchley (1969). He found that many patients could perform moderately well on the usual procedures of paper and pencil tasks and design copying with match sticks but would exhibit gross abnormalities when asked to assemble blocks into a three dimensional pattern. Often, in discussion, patients give no hints of impaired constructional ability, while, family members report that the patient has difficulty assembling familiar objects (Della Sala et al., 1987).

In response to these methodological problems, Benton (1968) developed and standardized a test which uses three block models. The first model uses six cubes, the second eight cubes, and the third fifteen cubes. The number and types of errors are recorded for each model. One hundred control subjects and an equal number of patients with brain disease were tested. The findings suggested that while constructional deficits may be associated with general mental impairment, mental impairment alone does not necessarily cause poor performance on this test. Twenty-five percent of the control group performed poorly on the test. Thus, constructional apraxia may appear in the absence of general cognitive impairment.

Two other evaluations utilize block construction tasks. The Boston Diagnostic Aphasia Examination (Goodglass & Kaplan, 1972) includes a block construction task as part of the battery. In these tests block constructions are reproduced from photographs. Barbara

Baum and her colleagues (1979) also included a block construction test in their Hemiplegic Evaluation.

The only study reported in the literature which compared performance across these measures (Benton, Goodglass & Kaplan, and Baum et al.) was conducted by Fall (1987). Fall administered all three constructional measures to a group of 24 subjects over the age of 70. The primary difference among the measures is the type of stimuli presented. She found that performance on constructional tasks is significantly affected by the type of stimuli used: the use of models resulted in significantly better performance than either schematic drawings or photographs.

The Relationship Between Constructional Apraxia and ADL

Most of the work examining the relationship of constructional apraxia to the performance of activities of daily living has been conducted with stroke patients. Lorenze and Cancro (1967) established a correlation between constructional ability and dressing performance in a group of 41 stroke patients. A drawing task was used to measure constructional deficits. The authors also studied grooming and feeding but did not find the same significant relationship with these variables as had been seen with dressing. Similarly, Williams (1967) observed a relationship between copying ability and upper extremity dressing in 136 stroke patients. Patients were asked to copy a series of three designs. Warren (1981) measured both constructional ability and body scheme disorders with 101 left and right CVA patients. Constructional ability was assessed by the Williams (1967) drawing task. The results indicated that both body scheme dysfunction and constructional apraxia were associated with impaired upper extremity dressing. However, body scheme deficits as measured by the Test of Body Scheme developed by MacDonald (1960) was a better overall predictor of dressing ability than was the constructional measure.

Baum and Hall (1981) studied both design copying and block construction in conjunction with upper extremity dressing in a group of 37 head injured adults. The Hemiplegic Evaluation developed at Massachusetts Rehabilitation Hospital (Baum et al., 1979) was used to determine graphic, two-dimensional and three-dimensional skill. Each of the constructional scores was significantly correlated with dressing ability at the .01 confidence level. Unlike Benton (1967) these authors found no difference in the performance of graphic, two-dimensional and three-dimensional praxis.

Constructional Apraxia and Alzheimer's Disease

There have been very few empirical studies of constructional apraxia in patients with global degenerative disease such as Alzheimer's disease. Mayer Gross (1935) described six patients with constructive apraxia. In five of these patients the illness became apparent at about age 50. All five complained of slowly increasing memory impairment, loss of interest in things around them and a tendency to lose their way in familiar surroundings. According to Mayer Gross, the men had failed in their profession and the women had given up housework. These symptoms are common indicators of the possible presence of senile dementia of the Alzheimer Type (SDAT). These patients also showed distinct difficulty with daily living tasks which required visuospatial skill such as putting on a shirt or tying a parcel.

Spatial disorientation in SDAT has not received much attention, nor has the relationship between spatial dysfunction and constructional apraxia been systematically explored. Relatively severe visuospatial deficits have been observed in some SDAT patients in a manner similar to the patterns of impaired language function (Cogan, 1985; Filley et al., 1986; Haxby et al., 1985). Similarly Baum et al. (1988) demonstrated that apraxia was related to, but distinguishable from language and measures of memory, orientation and learning. Recently, Henderson et al. (1989) found that spatial disorganization as measured by a visual constructive performance battery was predictive of problem wandering behaviors reported by caregivers. When these findings are considered in light of the anecdotal associations between constructional apraxia and problems of daily living reported in the clinical literature and the growing interest in parietal signs in SDAT the investigation of the presence of constructional apraxia warrants further attention.

METHODS

Subjects

The subjects for this study were participants in the Washington University Memory and Aging Project, a study of healthy aging and SDAT. All subjects were assessed with the Washington University Clinical Dementia Rating (CDR) (Berg, 1988). The CDR is a scale that rates dementia as absent, questionable, mild, moderate, or severe (CDR 0, 0.5, 1, 2, 3 respectively). The reliability and validity of the CDR rating has been established (Burke et al., 1988; Morris & McKeel, 1989) The present study involved 113 assessments of healthy intellectually preserved control subjects, 27 assessments of subjects with questionable dementia (CDR = 0.5), 34 assessments of subjects with mild dementia (CDR = 1), 29 assessments of subjects with moderate dementia (CDR = 2), and 52 assessments of subjects with severe dementia (CDR = 3). All participants were between 64 and 82 years of age at the time of enrollment. Although recruitment was not restricted by race, all participants were white; controls and subjects with SDAT did not differ in terms of education or social position. Subjects with potentially confounding neurologic, psychologic or medical disorders were not enrolled. All subjects met the NINCDS criteria for a diagnosis of dementia.

Measures

The 12 constructional apraxia test items are part of a larger 48 item test of manual apraxia. The Manual Apraxia Battery (Deuel, 1984) was developed to include items from several clinical tests of praxis (Sloan, 1955; Goodglass and Kaplan, 1972; DeRenzi et al., 1968, 1980). The test consists of four sections: (a) Imitation of Nonsense Gestures, (b) Pantomime on Command, (c) Use of Actual Objects, and (d) Colored Block Construction. The MAB has been determined to be an effective and sensitive measure of apraxia (Deuel et al., 1990). A scalar rating (0 = no impairment to 4 = severe impairment) is used for each item. The items within each subtest are summed to create subtest scores, all item scores are summed to create the total MAB score. For the purposes of this study the three geometric drawing items contained within the Use of Actual Objects scale have been combined with the nine block construction items to create a Constructional Apraxia scale. The geometric drawings were interspersed among the nine other items on the Use of Actual Objects scale. The subject was handed a pencil and a piece of paper and asked to draw a circle, a square, and a triangle. A three dimensional full scale model of each block construction was placed on the table in front of the subject. The subject was instructed to construct the model beside the model while it remained in full view, employing cubes from those loose on the table. One practice trial was given prior to the actual test items. Construction was timed. The block designs are presented in Figure 1.

The Katz ADL scale (Katz et al., 1963) was used to assess the caregiver's perception of the functional capacity of the patient. This 6 item questionnaire covers dressing, bathing, feeding, transfers, continence, and toileting. Each item is rated on a 4 point scale ranging from completely independent (0) to completely dependent (4). The score is the sum of the six ratings and ranges from 0 to 18. Both the apraxia battery and the Katz ADL scale were administered by an occupational therapist or a psychologist as part of the functional performance assessment battery.

Language function of the subjects was assessed using an Aphasia Battery that was derived from the Boston Diagnostic Aphasia Evaluation (Goodglass & Kaplan, 1983) and the Aphasia Language Performance Scales (Keenan & Brasseil, 1975). It includes subtests for expressive language, oral naming, reading comprehension, word discrimination, written naming, auditory comprehension, word discrimination and body part identification. Possible scores range from 0 (no errors) to 35 (total aphasia).

The Short Portable Mental Status Questionnaire (SPMSQ) developed by Pfeiffer (1974) as a brief measure of cognitive function was used to assess memory. This test consists of 10 items administered orally to the subject, and evaluates long term memory, information about current events, and the capacity to perform serial mental tasks. Its scores range from 0 (least affected) to 10 (most affected).

RESULTS

The means and standard deviations of the constructional apraxia scale are shown by CDR group in Table 1. As expected, the mean scores reveal an increase in constructional deficits as dementia pro-

FIGURE 1

COLORED BLOCK CONSTRUCTION DESIGNS

B - blue

G - green

O - orange

P - purple

R - red

Y - yellow

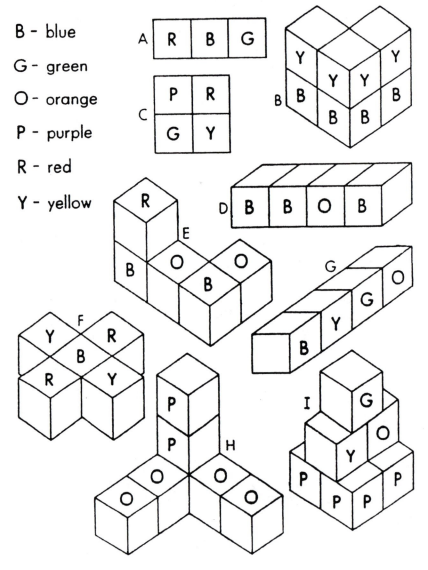

Table 1
Mean Constructional Apraxia Scores Shown By Stage of Dementia

Stage Of Dementia	N	Mean	SD	Range
Questionable (CDR 0.5)	28	5.68	5.58	0 - 19
Mild (CDR 1)	33	12.42	5.69	0 - 28
Moderate (CDR 2)	29	20.83	13.22	0 - 45
Severe (CDR 3)	51	43.27	9.53	0 - 48

gresses. Inspection of the ranges of total scores for each CDR group shows that there is considerable overlap across the groups. It is interesting to note that there are subjects in the moderate and severe stages of SDAT who were able to complete all 13 items without error. Correspondingly, there was one subject in the control group who demonstrated impaired performance on the construction items. A one way ANOVA examining differences across the CDR groups on the total constructional scale scores was significant ($F = 215.33$, $p < .0001$). Post hoc comparisons using the Duncan's Multiple Range Test indicated that there were no significant differences between the control, questionable and mild dementia groups. All three groups were significantly less impaired than the moderately and severely demented subjects.

The mean scores for the Katz ADL scale are presented by CDR group in Table 2. The scores for each of the ADL items are also shown in Table 2 as well as scores for the Aphasia Battery and the Short Portable Mental Status Questionnaire. Dressing performance was slightly more impaired at each stage of dementia than any of the other ADL items. The dressing score also shows an increase from a mean of 1.29 to a mean of 2.31 between the mild (CDR 1) and moderate (CDR 2) stage of dementia. The effects of SDAT were less obvious for Transfers. The Aphasia Battery scores increase slightly across the groups until the moderate stage, then there is a large increase in language dysfunction. The standard deviations for this measure are quite large in comparison to the mean scores, suggesting that the presence and extent of aphasia in the early stages of SDAT is highly variable.

In order to determine the relationship between constructional apraxia and the performance of basic activities of daily living a series of Pearson Product Moment correlation coefficients were computed for each stage of dementia. These findings are presented by CDR group in Table 3.

Prior research has raised the issue of the association between language function and different types of apraxia. This factor has been cited (Benton, 1967) as particularly important when the subject is asked to draw a geometric figure by the examiner. Persons with SDAT also have significant memory impairment which may limit their ability to perform constructional tasks if the task requires short

Table 2

Performance on Activities of Daily Living, Aphasia and
Memory Measures Shown By Stage of Dementia

Variable	Questionable Mean ± SD	Mild Mean ± SD	Moderate Mean ± SD	Severe Mean± SD
Katz ADL Score	6.64± 1.65	6.69±1.33	9.10± 2.88	13.31± 2.70
Bathing	1.11± 0.47	1.24±0.57	1.93± 0.92	2.83± 0.44
Dressing	1.17± 0.51	1.29±0.63	2.31± 0.89	2.86± 0.48
Toileting	1.05± 0.23	1.04±0.21	1.31± 0.54	2.05± 0.62
Transfers	1.00± 0.00	1.02±0.15	1.07±0.26	1.37± 0.55
Continence	1.06± 0.24	1.07±0.25	1.34±0.61	2.32± 0.75
Feeding	1.06± 0.24	1.02±0.15	1.14±0.35	1.95± 0.74
Aphasia Score	1.32± 1.65	3.21±3.70	8.59±7.70	27.51± 7.04
SPMSQ	1.96± 1.79	5.41±2.40	8.31±1.58	9.78± 0.59

Table 3
Correlations Between Constructional Apraxia and Katz ADL
Scale Items Shown BY Stage of Dementia

Variable	Questionable	Mild	Moderate	Severe
Total Katz Score	- 0.15	0.00	0.62 ***	0.15
Bathing	- 0.10	-0.21	0.59 ***	0.07
Dressing	- 0.32	0.37*	0.62 ***	0.08
Toileting	- 0.07	0.01	0.45 *	0.16
Transfers	0.00	0.00	0.21	0.28
Continence	- 0.07	0.01	0.50 **	0.12
Feeding	- 0.07	0.00	0.35	0.20

* p< .05
** p< .01
***p< .001

term memory. In order to determine the differential contribution of both memory and language a series of correlation coefficients were computed by CDR group. The Aphasia battery was not significantly correlated with constructional performance in the questionable and mild SDAT subjects. These same results were seen in terms of memory performance as assessed by the SPMSQ. Significant correlations were found for both aphasia and memory in the moderate dementia group (CDR 2), the correlation coefficients were r = .67, and r = .52 for aphasia and memory respectively. A different pattern was observed in the severe dementia group (CDR 3). In this group, the aphasia battery scores were correlated with constructional performance (r = .66) but the association between the SPMSQ and constructional apraxia was substantially diminished (r = .17). The correlations of the aphasia battery were slightly higher than those of the SPMSQ. These findings suggest that there is a consistent language effect present in constructional tasks of this type.

When the individual ADL items were examined, the constructional apraxia score was always more highly correlated with ADL performance than were aphasia or memory.

DISCUSSION

The results of this study clearly demonstrate that constructional deficits are present in some patients at the very early stages of dementia. While it is commonly accepted that apraxic deficits of all types are seen in SDAT patients, most investigators have not had access to patients in the earliest stages of the disease, and thus have concluded that apraxia is an end stage rather than early phenomenon. The practical consequence of these findings is tremendous, both in terms of patient functioning and caregiver stress. The results of this study substantiate the need for early assessment and intervention to assist both the patient and his family in addressing functional loss. Family members often assume that ADL difficulties encountered in the early stages of SDAT are attitudinal rather than neurological in nature. They may feel that the patient is seeking attention and that he/she could more than adequately perform the tasks if they felt like it. Intervention is more likely to yield successful results if these deficits are recognized in the early stages of SDAT. Many of the techniques developed to assist patients with other types of neurological deficits (i.e., strokes and head injuries) to address constructional problems could be adapted to the needs of Alzheimer's patients and their families.

It is also important to recognize that there is tremendous variability in SDAT patients. For example, the findings of this study demonstrate that it is possible to be severely demented, with virtually no memory, and still be able to successfully complete all of the items in the constructional apraxia battery without committing any errors. These findings are consistent with results reported by Benton et al. (1984) who found that not all patients with similar lesions presented with constructional deficits, as well as with a number of other investigations of patients with SDAT (Martin et al., 1986; Neary et al., 1986). These studies have shown that there is considerable heterogeneity among persons with SDAT such that persons within the same stage of dementia may show different areas of preservation of cognitive skills.

The dressing scores on the Katz ADL scale suggest that problems with dressing are an early and persistent problem in persons with SDAT. The mean scores for dressing show that this area is more impaired than other ADL skills across all stages of dementia. The results of this study imply that dressing and bathing progressively decline across the CDR groups, while other skills such as feeding and transfers are stable until the severe (CDR 3) stage.

The relationship between constructional apraxia and dressing observed in stroke patients (Williams, 1967) and persons with closed head injuries (Baum & Hall, 1981) was also obtained in this sample of persons with SDAT. At the questionable, mild and moderate stages the highest correlations were generated between the dressing variable and constructional apraxia. The correlations for the CDR 3 (severe dementia) group are difficult to interpret since many of these subjects are so severely impaired that they only engage in the most basic of functional activities such as transferring from chair to bed, and chewing and swallowing food. Thus, the focus of these findings should be on the less significantly impaired subjects.

RECOMMENDATIONS

The relationship between the different types of constructional skill (i.e., design copying and block construction) and ADL performance was not examined in this study. This relationship warrants further investigation. Until these relationships are clearly understood, therapists should include all three areas, graphic, two-dimensional, and three-dimensional tasks in their assessment of constructional deficits, as opposed to reliance on tests which assess only one or two of these domains.

REFERENCES

Baum, B., & Hall, K.M. (1981). Relationship between constructional praxis and dressing in the head injured adult. *American Journal of Occupational Therapy*, 35, 438-442.

Baum, B., Levine, M., Lonigan, M., Siev, E., Silverman, E., Solet, J., & Wall, N. (1979). *Hemiplegic Evaluation*. Boston: Massachusetts Rehabilitation Hospital, Occupational Therapy Department.

Baum, C., Edwards, D., Leavitt, K., Grant, E., & Deuel, R. (1988). Performance components in senile dementia of the Alzheimer type: Motor planning, language and memory. *Occupational Therapy Journal of Research*, 8, 356-368.

Benton, A. (1967). Constructional apraxia and the minor hemisphere. *Conferences in Neurology*, 29, 1-16.

Benton, A. (1968). Differential behavioral effects in frontal lobe disease. *Neuropsychologia*, 6, 53-60.

Berg, L. (1988). Clinical Dementia Rating (CDR). *Psychopharmacology Bullitin*, 24, 637-639.

Burke, W., Miller, J., Rubin, E. & Morris, J. (1988). Reliability of the Washington University Clinical Dementia Rating (CDR). *Annals of Neurology*, 24, 17-22.

Cogan, D. (1985). Visual disturbances with focal progressive dementing disease. *American Journal of Opthalmology*, 100, 68-72.

Critchley, M. (1971). *The Parietal Lobes*. Hafner, New York.

Della Sala, S., Lucelli, F., & Spinnler, H. (1987). Ideomotor apraxia in patients with dementia of the Alzheimer type. *Journal of Neurology*, 243, 91-93.

DeRenzi, E. & Luccelli, F. (1988). Ideational apraxia. *Brain*, 111, 1173-1185.

DeRenzi, E., Vignolo, L. & Pieczuro, A. (1968). Ideational apraxia: A quantitative study. *Neuropsychologia*, 6, 41-52.

DeRenzi, E., Motti, F. & Nichelli, P. (1980). Imitating gestures: A quantitative approach to ideomotor apraxia. *Archives of Neurology*, 37, 6-10.

Deuel, R., Feely, C., & Bonskowski, C. (1984). Manual apraxia in learning diabled children. (abstr.) *Annals of Neurology*, 16, 388.

Deuel, R., Edwards, D. & Baum, C. (1990). Properties of apraxia test items that distinguish early states of dementia. (abstr.) *Annals of Neurology*, 21.

Fall, C. (1987). Comparing ways of measuring constructional praxis in the well elderly. *American Journal of Occupational Therapy*, 41, 500-504.

Filley, C., Kelley, J., & Heaton, R. (1986). Neuropsychologic features of early and late onset Alzheimer's disease. *Archives of Neurology*, 43, 574-576.

Goodglass, H. & Kaplan, E. (1983). The assesment of aphasia and related disorders. *2nd ed.* Philadelphia: Lea & Febiger.

Haxby, J., Duara, R., Grady, C., Cutler, N., & Rappoport, S. (1985). Relations between neuropsychological and cerebral assymetries in early Alzheimer's disease. *Journal of Cerebral Blood Flow and Metabolism*, 5, 193-200.

Henderson, V., Mack, W. & Williams, B. (1989). Spatial disorientation in Alzheimer's disease. *Archives of Neurology*, 46, 391-394.

Katz, S., Ford, A., Maskowitz, R. & Jackson, B. (1963). Studies of illness in the aged: A standardized measure of biological and psychological function. *Journal of the American Medical Association*, 135, 75-86.

Kleist, K. (1934). *Gehirnpathologie*. Barth, Leipzig.

Lorenze, E., & Cancro, R. (1962). Dysfunction in visual perception with hemiplegia: Its relation to activities of daily living. *Archives of Physical Medicine and Rehabilitation*, 43, 514-517.

MacDonald, J. (1960). An investigation of body scheme in adults with cerebral vascular accidents. *American Journal of Occupational Therapy*, 14, 75-79.

Mayer-Gross, W. (1935). Some observations on apraxia. *Proceedings of the Royal Society of Medicine*, 28, 1203-1212.

Morris, J., McKeel, D., Fulling, K., Torack, R. & Berg, L. (1988). Validation of clinical diagnostic criteria for Alzheimer's disease. *Archives of Neurology*, 45, 31-32.32

Pfeiffer, E. (1975). A short portable mental status questionnaire for the assessment of organic brain defect in elderly patients. *Journal of the American Geriatric Society*, 23, 433-441.

Sloan, W. (1948). *The Lincoln Adaptation of the Oseretsky Tests*. Lincoln IL: Lincoln State School and Colony.

van der Horst (1934). Constructive Apraxia: Some views on the conception of space. *Journal of Nervous and Mental Disease*, 80, 645-650.

Williams, N. (1967). Correlation between copying ability and dressing activities in hemiplegia. *American Journal of Physical Medicine*, 46, 1332-1340.

Helping Those with Dementia
to Live at Home:
An Educational Series
for Caregivers

Danielle N. Butin, MPH, OTR

SUMMARY. A four part educational series has been developed at
The New York Hospital-Cornell Medical Center, Westchester Division, for caregivers of persons with dementia living at home. The
four consecutive sessions provide caregivers with practical solutions
in home safety, activities of daily living, adaptive equipment, leisure, communication, and accessing community resources. The goal
of the series is to promote effective caregiving strategies and to improve the quality of life for the person with dementia living at home.

Approximately 10% of all people over age 65 have clinically
significant intellectual impairments, and half of this cohort have
dementia (Beck, 1982). The two main subgroups of dementia are
Alzheimer's Disease and Multi-Infarct Dementia. Alzheimer's Disease is the most common, and is characterized by the progressive
deterioration of intellectual functioning. Multi-Infarct Dementia
results from a series of mini-strokes that can affect memory and
other cortical functions (Mace & Rabins, 1981). Other definitions
of dementia include a progressive failure of the patient in all activities of daily living, failure of all cognitive functions and disruption
in the personality structure. This slow unraveling of self can lead to

Danielle N. Butin is Occupational Therapist in the Geriatric Services Division
at The New York Hospital-Cornell Medical Center, Westchester Division. She
has developed and implemented educational programs for caregivers and
healthcare professionals working with demented patients. Address correspondence to the author at 21 Bloomingdale Road, White Plains, NY 10605.

physical deterioration and even to psychotic symptoms of delusions and hallucinations (Roth & Myers, 1975).

The tremendous task of caregiving has slowly gained recognition and service intervention from the health care system. The complicated and conflictual roles of the "sandwich generation" are being taken seriously, and are addressed as life events warranting intervention. Adult children often have mixed responses to caregiving and to the responsibility of caring for an impaired older parent (Teusink & Mahler, 1985). While social workers are most commonly identified for the leadership of caregiver groups, occupational therapists are being recognized as having crucial roles in teaching families ways to manage relatives for success at home. Occupational Therapists have published on adaptive strategies for the patient with dementia (Butin, 1989, Griffin, 1990, Levy, 1986, Levy, 1989, McDonald, 1985, Zgola, 1989), yet little has been recorded on the application of principles used in clinical practice to educate family members. Traditional caregiver support groups succeed at processing feelings and attitudes, but may lack a pragmatic "how to" approach for dealing with everyday problems.

At The New York Hospital, Cornell Medical Center-Westchester Division, a four-part caregiver series has been implemented to assist those caring for a person with dementia in the community. It is believed that in order for caregivers to succeed in areas of home management and safety, they need to understand dementia and how to respond most effectively to patients' behaviors, while also becoming aware of available community resources (Skinner & Jordan, 1989). The four part caregiver series was designed to offer practical assistance to caregivers and to foster safe and qualitative functioning for the impaired person at home.

The series is available to family members, friends and home health aides caring for patients hospitalized at The New York Hospital. Referral to the group is made by the occupational therapist on each unit. Since the series is ongoing, families can enter the program at any point, and consecutive attendance is not mandatory. It seems most important to provide a flexible and easily accessible forum for caregivers who are usually quite stressed and overwhelmed by the prospect of having the patient at home. The series has also been offered for time limited periods at local community centers, and home health agencies.

The series objectives are that the participants will:

1. Learn practical aspects of the condition and how it affects daily functioning.
2. Learn the environmental adaptations necessary to safely manage their family member at home.
3. Learn adaptive strategies to promote increased independence in all activities of daily living.
4. Become aware of adaptive equipment options that aid in mealtime, dressing, bathing and toileting safety.
5. Learn adaptive activity interventions to facilitate meaningful and appropriate leisure involvements.
6. Learn methods for communicating effectively with the patient.
7. Receive resource materials and catalogs to better access and use existing community services.

SESSION ONE: OVERVIEW OF DEMENTIA AND HOME SAFETY

An overview of the progressive illness of dementia is reviewed. Participants are encouraged to understand the individuality of the disease and how differently patients may function. Changes in overall function are presented, with respect to mental status, visual-perceptual skills, activities of daily living and leisure involvements. Caregivers are presented with methods and strategies for adapting the home for safety.

As the disease progresses a deterioration is noted in certain areas of emotional functioning. It is important for families to recognize these changes as part of the disease process, and not as acts of volition. A list of common changes is shared with families, because these changes frequently require early recognition for treatment and some symptom remission.

Mental Status Changes

ORIENTATION: The person may not know where he/she is, and may become unaware of time. Eventually, the person may have difficulties recognizing his/her family, friends or self.

MEMORY: The person is unable to retain short-term information or recall recent events. The person may ask the same questions repetitively, because he/she cannot remember asking questions or receiving a response.

SAFETY AWARENESS AND JUDGEMENT: The ability to recognize danger or unsafe situations is impaired. The person is generally quite distractible and shows poor judgment with a lack of caution.

DEPRESSION: In the beginning stages of the disease, the person may show signs of a clinical depression. They are acutely aware of the changes, and therefore more prone to significant reactions. If the following symptoms appear, then it is important to seek out treatment: decreased sleep, decreased appetite, irritability, sadness or wish to be dead. As the dementing illness progresses, it becomes more difficult for the person to verbalize feelings, and vegetative symptoms need careful observation and recognition.

DELUSIONS: Fearful and suspicious thoughts may appear. They are false beliefs that seem very real to the person suffering with these thoughts. He/she may accuse family members of stealing, or plotting against him/her.

HALLUCINATIONS: The person may see or hear things that are not real.

Families are educated about the seriousness of the three psychiatric symptoms (depression, delusions and hallucinations) and how they each warrant a thorough evaluation for treatment. Caregivers learn the significance of these behaviors, and geriatric psychiatry referrals are made available for all group members. Geriatric psychiatrists seem best trained to comprehensively treat the psychiatric symptoms of medically and socially complicated patients.

Families also benefit from learning about visual-perceptual changes, and how this affects one's ability to understand and integrate information. It is frequently difficult for the demented person to accommodate to fluorescent or dim lighting, bold prints, or multi-colored rooms. The following modifications make functioning easier for the demented patient with visual-perceptual difficulties:

Visual-Perceptual Modifications

1. Solid colored walls
2. Solid colored floors or carpet
3. Solid colored sheets with different colored spread.
4. Colored toilet seat cover
5. Colored waste basket in bathroom
6. Red on white signs for rooms
7. Plates on table different color from placemat.

For families, it is also essential to understand the need for overall safety in the home. This session ends with one part of a slide show lecture "Adaptive Strategies for the Alzheimer's Patient" (Butin, 1987), that emphasizes all areas of functioning for the demented patient. The slide show provides visual displays of the recommended strategies. Families are given a home safety checklist and are encouraged to review potential modifications.

Home Safety Checklist

1. Use night lights in bedroom, bathroom and hallway
2. Remove scatter rugs
3. Install smoke alarms
4. Change locks on front and back doors
5. Remove locks from bedroom and bathrooms
6. Lock up all medications, cleaning fluids, sharp objects, and other dangerous items
7. Install detachable oven and stove knobs
8. Turn down hot water temperature
9. Avoid rearranging furniture
10. Use non-skid wax on polished floors
11. Place a safety gate at the top of the stairs
12. Avoid cluttered shelves, replace with family photographs.

SESSION TWO: ACTIVITIES OF DAILY LIVING AND ADAPTIVE EQUIPMENT

An overview of all activities of daily living is provided. Family members are introduced to adaptive equipment used to increase safety and independence in bathing, toileting, dressing and eating. A demonstration of this adaptive equipment and of transfer techniques is provided, in conjunction with the slide-show demonstration.

Since a significant number of falls occur at night, one must give special attention to the bathroom to assure safety. The importance of a professional and thorough home evaluation is stressed. Trained to assess equipment needs and to make precise measurements, occupational therapists can help families locate appropriate adaptive devices. Additionally, occupational therapists who have had experience working with cognitively impaired patients can be especially helpful to caregivers in ways to creatively approach these patients' specialized needs. During the training session, caregivers receive a complete introduction to adaptive equipment, and a full explanation of its appropriate use and application. Equipment reviewed includes: toilet grab bars, elevated toilet seats, padded tub seat or bench, hand held shower spray, and shower grab bars. The following adaptations are also discussed and recommended when appropriate:

Bathroom Modifications

1. Non-skid colorful surface on bottom of tub
2. Use colorful flower over drain of tub
3. Avoid leaving soap on sink
4. Sign reminding patient to flush the toilet
5. Use colorful toilet paper and toilet seat cover.

The colorful toilet seat and paper may help the patient with figure ground difficulties. Male patients frequently urinate on the toilet seat lid. The colorful seat alerts the patient to the need to raise the cover. Patients are often frightened of bathing, and become resistive and very anxious during this activity. Family members are encouraged to provide environmental adaptations that promote a sense of comfort and security during this activity. Non-skid stickers on the bottom of the tub, with a plastic flower covering the drain has also worked effectively. Patients with dementia frequently view the tub as a bottomless pit and claim that the drain will pull them under. These simple adaptations have proven quite effective in allaying their fears. For patients who simply fear the sound of running water, some plan for systematic desensitization is appropriate. The caregiver begins by helping the patient tolerate the sound of running water in the bathroom, and then slowly works towards the shower.

Dressing is another area of daily living activities stressed in the caregiver group, since sequencing purposeful and logical motor acts is difficult for persons with dementia. Families are encouraged to use specific cuing for optimal independence. Clothing should be simple to don and doff. A list of adaptive clothing manufacturers is provided. Families are encouraged to offer their patient one or two choices from a repertoire of wraparound or elastic band skirts for women, and sweatsuits with velcro fastenings on pants for men. Adaptive devices used to help in dressing are often too complicated for demented patients to understand. Instead, families are encouraged to identify the specific time or activity that prove difficult during dressing, and provide cues only during those instances.

Like other activities of daily living, mealtime can be overwhelming for patients with dementia and for their caregivers, An array of different color and size platters, plates, and utensils is too visually stimulating and can add to perceptual difficulties. Therefore, caregivers are encouraged to keep mealtime activities as simple as possible. First, participation in family style meals, when large platters of food are passed around the table, should be eliminated. It is generally advised that pre-seasoned, pre-cut food be provided to be eaten with a soup spoon or fork. However, since abilities and preferences vary, adaptive equipment is demonstrated during the class session to offer alternatives for promoting independence. For example, plate guards can be helpful for controlling plate contents, and spill proof cups can reduce accidents with fluids. For individuals who have limited grasp or tremulous hands, other adaptive utensils are presented. Caregivers are encouraged to use the following recommendations:

Mealtime Suggestions

1. Gently remind the person of what he/she is eating
2. Cue the person to open the mouth and to chew
3. Observe the person to ensure that they swallow, and provide cues if necessary.
4. Encourage the person to eat at his/her own pace.
5. Cue the person to drink liquids during the meal.

Caregivers should also consider the adaptive equipment resources and vendors listed (Appendix).

SESSION THREE: LEISURE ACTIVITIES AND COMMUNICATION

Class members are given an overview of different methods of communication, and ways to adapt activities. Caregivers learn helpful interactive strategies, and how to apply these to meaningful leisure pursuits. Ideas of how to adapt past leisure interests to present levels of functioning are presented, and resources for mail-ordering supplies for activities at home are distributed.

Successful communication is essential if the person with dementia is to maintain a sense of connectedness and belonging. Caregivers benefit from hearing specific ways which have been used successfully and which may be helpful alternatives in moments of tremendous frustration. Caregivers benefit from trying new communication strategies, and/or problem solving specific problem situations within the group.

Communication Strategies

1. Address person directly in front of him/her
2. Speak calmly and clearly
3. Be concise
4. Repeat when the person is not able to follow the conversation
5. Simplify conversations or words used if the person does not understand
6. Ask the person how he/she feels

7. Verbally recognize discomfort, and redirect if necessary
8. Always listen to what the person is saying.

Effective communication that produces clear and simple understanding is important if any meaningful activities are to be undertaken. If families can master useful communication strategies, they can begin to facilitate involvement in activities.

Unfortunately, activity suggestions frequently are doomed before they are ever introduced, because families are so disheartened by the deterioration they see, that using simplified activity is perceived as childlike and infantilizing. It is the occupational therapist's challenge to help families understand the importance of keeping the person active physically and mentally. Therapists can then perform activity analyses with families and support their role in maintaining levels of function and providing a sense of accomplishment. Activity education must respond to feelings of disappointment, while building up a resource of optimistic and pleasurable activities for the family to use in interacting with their patient. If a collaborative effort between the patient and family is to take place, then caregivers must understand the whole process before planning or participating in activities. Activities are interesting and intriguing if they are presented with enthusiasm and a sense of purpose. One way to show caregivers the impact of having unstructured time with no activities for their patient, is to ask them to imagine a week without their date book, and to exaggerate that experience by being in a state of confusion. Families identify with the exercise and learn that this feeling contributes to agitation, wandering and increased irritability. Cognitively impaired adults can still engage in meaningful activities and benefit from their outcomes, experience joy and derive a sense of accomplishment. Families need assistance in identifying the right functional level/need/activity match for their loved one. Creativity, flexibility and risk taking are encouraged and valued in the group. They are encouraged to break down individualized meaningful activities into simple step directions. Caregivers list purposeful activities used in the past and learn to brainstorm adaptations for current use. A sample list of adapted leisure activities is provided during the group.

Adapted Leisure Activities

Homemaking: 1. Assisting in bedmaking
               2. Hanging, sorting, folding laundry
               3. Matching socks (two colors)
               4. Dusting or sweeping
               5. Drying dishes
               6. Sorting spoons and forks
               7. Assisting in setting the table
               8. Assisting in cold food preparation
               9. Cutting out coupons for food shopping

Business: 1. Sorting coins (two types)
               2. Stuffing and stamping envelopes
               3. Sorting large pieces of paper
               4. Sorting pens and pencils
               5. Arranging canceled checks.

Similarly, if a patient has enjoyed music in the past, then he may find satisfaction from singing along to old favorite songs on the stereo, listening to seasonal music for reality orientation, or playing games associated with music.

The methods outlined can be applied to all areas of interest, such as sports, gardening, art. Specific vendors have developed and sell ideas and kits for the memory impaired. Families are given an extensive resource list for activities. Two manufacturers have provided ideas with exceptional opportunities for meaningful involvement of memory impaired persons. Cross Creek Productions have test marketed all of their products, and offer colorful, large and intriguing puzzles and games. Visuo-spatial games in particular prove an enjoyable package of options. Patients enjoy these activities, which are highly recommended to families. Elder Games, another vendor, has developed a series of group games for patients and their families. These games promote family involvement in a leisure activity adapted for success of the confused person. Elder Trivia is one of their products, and provides long term memory questions consisting of simple retrievable facts.

During this third caregiver session, an exercise program is demonstrated for families, and they are encouraged to duplicate it each morning with their patient. Families are given a hand-out detailing exercises with instructions to play favorite music. The activity ends with balloon volleyball. Throughout this session, the rationale for activities is continually emphasized, because it is the foundation for all creative efforts.

Posting a daily schedule on the refrigerator is comforting to them since these persons have difficulties with unstructured time. Breaking up the day's events into simple increments provides a reassuring and meaningful structure. A sample schedule is illustrated:

Sunday, December 3, 1990

    8 AM EAT BREAKFAST
    9 AM EXERCISE
    10 AM FOOD SHOPPING
    11 AM UNPACK GROCERIES
    12 PM PREPARE AND EAT LUNCH

This format should be followed every day from morning to evening. The caregiver should begin each day with discussion of the schedule, and explain each incremental event to the patient. A slide show accompanies this session and further illustrates schedules and adapted activities for family guidance.

SESSION FOUR: ACCESSING COMMUNITY RESOURCES

An overview of all essential community resources for persons with dementia is provided in this session. Time is allowed for caregivers to identify specific areas of concern (home safety, ADL, or leisure), and to use the group for problem solving. Each group member receives a folder of all local resources that might address their needs.

An explanation of the concept of continuum of services is provided during the final session. How to access local home health agencies is explained, and information brochures from three local agencies are discussed. A full explanation of the rationale and routines of day care programs follows a review of local resources. Respite services are reviewed, along with the benefits of belonging to a local support group. The criteria for psychiatric hospitalization are explained as well as options for outpatient care. Because the overall objective of the series is to promote and facilitate community living for as long as possible, resources to aid nursing home placement are only briefly addressed.

In the final session, caregivers are encouraged to share their specific problems, and/or to share successful strategies that others could use. Questions have included such difficulties as buckling pants, helping an angry person to eat, and ways of progressing from sponge bathing to using a shower seat. Caregivers frequently share their methods with one another. The occupational therapist adds recommendations.

SUMMARY

A four-part educational series has been successfully offered to caregivers of persons with dementia at home. Occupational therapists play a strong, vital role in teaching caregivers the creativity, adaptation and confidence necessary for the everyday activities of caring for a family member with dementia. Practical solutions offer support to families, and facilitate greater skill in problem solving and the utilization of adaptive strategies. Teaching the process of activity analysis enables caregivers of demented persons to succeed in tasks that had been previously overwhelming.

REFERENCES

Beck, J.C., Benson, D.F., Scheibel, A.B., Spar, J.E., Rubenstein, L.D. (1982). Dementia in the elderly: the silent epidemic. *Annals of Internal Medicine*, 97, 231-241.

Butin, D. (1987). Adaptive strategies for the Alzheimer's patient. *Slide Show Lecture*.

Butin, D. (1989). Helping Alzheimer's patients live at home. *The Senior Patient*, November/December, 72-79.

Griffin, R. M. (1990). *Protocols for adapting activities to the changing needs of people with dementia*. Baltimore, MD: Chess Publications.

Levy, L.L. (1986). A practical guide to the care of the Alzheimer's disease victim: the cognitive disability perspective. *Topics in Geriatric Rehabilitation*, 1,(2), 16-26.

Levy, L.L. (1989). Activity adaptation in rehabilitation of the physically and cognitively disabled aged. *Topics in Geriatric Rehabilitation*, 4,(4), 53-66.

Mace, N.L. & Rabins, P.V. (1981). *The 36 hour day*. Baltimore, MD: Johns Hopkins Press.

MacDonald, K.C. (1986). Occupational therapy approaches to treatment of dementia patients. *Physical & Occupational Therapy in Geriatrics*, 4 (2), 61-72.

Roth, M. & Myers, O.H. (1975). The diagnosis of dementia. In T. Silverstone & B. Barraclough (Ed.) *Contemporary Psychiatry*, 9, England: Headley Brothers.

Skinner, P.V. & Jordan, D. (1989). Home management of the patient with Alzheimer's disease. *Home Healthcare Nurse*, 7 (1), 23-27.

Teusink, J.P. & Mahler, S. (1984). Helping families cope with Alzheimer's disease. *Journal of Hospital and Community Psychiatry*, 35, 152-156.

Zgola, Jitka. (1989). *Doing things*. Baltimore, MD: Johns Hopkins Press.

APPENDIX

RESOURCE GUIDE

ACTIVITIES

Cross Creek Productions
Amenia, New York

Elder Games
Rockville, Maryland 20852

BiFolkl Kits
Madison, Wisconsin 53703

Worldwide Games
Colchester, Connecticut 06415

CLOTHING

Sears Home Health Care Catalog
White Plains, New York 10601

Exceptionally Yours
Newtonville, MA 02160

Techni Flair
Cotter, Arkansas 72626

Geri-Wear Clothing
South Bend, Indiana 46624

Comfortably Yours
Maywood, New Jersey 07607

ACTIVITIES OF DAILY LIVING

Ways and Means-The Capability Collection
Romules, Michigan 48174

Solutions
Portland, Oregon 97228-6878

Fred Sammons-BEOK
Brookfield, Illinois 60513

Enrichments
Hinsdale, Illinois 60521

In-Home Interventions for Persons with Alzheimer's Disease and Their Caregivers

Jon Pynoos, PhD
Russell J. Ohta, PhD

SUMMARY. A multi-disciplinary pilot research project assessed the needs of persons with Alzheimer's disease and their caregivers in the home, identified target areas for intervention, and implemented specific caregiver-selected interventions. An evaluation of the pilot project indicated that a majority of the interventions that caregivers considered initially effective still worked approximately seven to nine months later. This relative stability of initially-effective interventions continued for many caregivers despite progressive declines in the functioning of the persons with Alzheimer's. The results also suggest the importance of enhancing the effectiveness of interventions when first introduced.

Key words: Dementia, Caregiving, Community-based

Jon Pynoos is the United Parcel Service Foundation Associate Professor of Gerontology, Public Policy and Urban Planning, and Director, Program in Policy and Services Research, Andrus Gerontology Center, University of Southern California, Los Angeles, CA 90089-0191.

Russell J. Ohta was formerly Director, the Caring Home Program. Currently he is Partner, Southwest Geriatric Consultation Services, 8415 N. 17th Place, Phoenix, AZ 85020.

This program was supported by grants from the Andrus Foundation of the American Association of Retired Persons and the Alzheimer's Disease Program of the California Department of Health Services, with additional support from the Tingstad Alzheimer's Disease Research Fund. The authors wish to gratefully acknowledge the contribution of the following individuals to the program: Eileen Haller, MSG, Sandra Hattori, MSG, OTR, Evelyn Cohen, MA, and Claire Lucas, MSG.

The home is the major setting in which care is provided to persons with Alzheimer's disease. Most persons who have Alzheimer's disease are cared for at home by their families for the majority of their illness. The Alzheimer's Association estimates that six times as many persons live in the community as in nursing homes (Alzheimer's Disease and Related Disorders Association, 1985).

Considerable attention has been directed to assisting caregivers with the monumental task they face in providing care at home. The programs generally focus on educational/training materials for caregivers (e.g., caregiver seminars and pamphlets), emotional support (e.g., caregiver support groups), respite (e.g., adult day health care), and/or direct in-home care of the patient (e.g., home health services). Although not as widely recognized, efforts have also been directed to making the physical characteristics of the home environment as conducive as possible to the care of a person who has Alzheimer's disease (Kern, 1986; Pynoos and Cohen, 1989; Pynoos, Cohen, and Lucas, 1988; Skolaski-Pellitteri, 1984; Zgola, 1990).

This paper describes a pilot research project designed to better understand the role of the home environment in the care of persons with Alzheimer's disease. The project consisted of: (1) an assessment of the level of functioning of the person with the disease and problems experienced by the caregiver; (2) an independent assessment of the home environment; (3) identification of target areas for intervention; (4) the implementation of specific caregiver-selected interventions; and (5) an evaluation of intervention effectiveness. The project paid particular attention to the environmental aspects of caregiving in the home, and the adaptations or modifications to the home which might be of benefit to the caregiver.

METHOD

The study was conducted in two stages. In Stage one, 25 persons with Alzheimer's disease and their caregivers were selected. They were obtained from local support groups, adult day care centers, and other agencies in the area, as well as through newspaper advertisements and press releases. In order to participate, the caregiver needed to be the primary care provider for the person with Alzheimer's disease and be residing in the same home. The person with Alzheimer's disease must have had a complete medical examination within the previous six months (including blood and urine testing), a complete neurological examination (including either a CT scan, PET scan or MRI), must not have been bedridden, and must not have been severely impaired on four or more of the remaining activities of daily living (bathing, feeding, dressing, grooming, transfer, toileting, continence care).

Demographic information about the person with Alzheimer's and the caregiver, along with caregiver reports of the patient's ADL and IADL functioning were obtained by telephone. This was followed by a home visit during which the frequency of problems, and the caregiver's reactions to them, were surveyed by a clinical gerontologist. This survey involved the use of the Problems and Barriers Survey, a 44-item instrument developed for this program (expanding the 29-item Memory and Behavior Problems Checklist of Zarit et al., 1980 and Zarit, 1982). An independent assessment and photography of the home environment was also conducted by an occupational therapist, using the Home Environmental Assessment Checklist also developed for this project.

After all information was obtained for each participant, the project field team, which consisted of the clinical gerontologist, the occupational therapist and a psychologist met to review the information. Based upon the level of functioning of the person with Alzheimer's disease, caregiver-experienced problems and reactions, and assessment of the home environment, the team identified and developed priorities for what it considered to be the most critical problems faced by each caregiver and generated a set of interventions for dealing with each problem. This list of problems and proposed interventions was then presented to the caregiver for consideration and feedback. The caregiver selected those problems which he or she wanted addressed and the desired mode of intervention. Up to one hundred dollars was provided by the project for changes. The interventions were then implemented by the project team at no charge to the caregiver.

In Stage two, caregivers were contacted seven months later concerning their ability and willingness to be involved in a follow-up study. By that time, the sample of participants had shrunk to 12

caregivers owing to eight hospitalizations and/or institutionaliza-
tions of persons with Alzheimer's disease, four caregivers who declined to continue and one caregiver whom the researchers could
not contact.

The 12 caregivers who received program interventions and were
available for follow-up consisted of 7 women and 5 men, 11 of
whom were spouses of persons with Alzheimer's disease and 1 of
whom was an adult child. The average age of the caregivers was
70.8 years, and they had been providing care for an average of 40.1
months. The average age of the person with Alzheimer's was 77.3
years, and their activities of daily living (ADL) scores averaged
16.9 (possible range of 8-48, with higher scores indicating greater
impairment) while their instrumental activities of daily living
(IADL) scores averaged 37.2 (possible range of 8-46, with higher
scores indicating greater impairment).

ANALYSIS OF DATA

The data from Stage one of the project indicated that caregivers
experienced a number of environmentally related problems and reported that many of the interventions made it easier and safer to
provide care (Pynoos and Ohta, 1988). A total of 29 problems had
been addressed for the 12 caregivers interviewed in the second
stage. There were single instances of interventions for the problems
of engaging in behavior that is potentially dangerous to self and
using stairs. There were two instances of interventions for the problems of forgetting what day it is, getting lost outside the home,
losing/misplacing things, and feeding self, and three for the problems of long periods of inactivity, toileting, and continence care.
The dominant problem addressed by the program was that of bathing, for which there were ten instances of interventions. Chart 1
lists the caregiver-selected interventions implemented for the various problems.

Data reflecting the effectiveness of interventions are presented in
Table 1.

The interviews revealed that, for 19 of the 29 problems addressed
(or 66% of the total), interventions were evaluated by the caregivers
as having been effective when first introduced. Furthermore, inter-

Chart 1

Project Interventions Selected by Caregivers

Problem	Interventions
Behavior dangerous to self	Non-electric shaver
Using stairs	Handrail
Forgetting the day	Reality orientation board
Getting lost outside	Identification bracelet
Losing/misplacing things	Locked security box
Feeding self	Partitioned plate, scoop dish, spork
Inactivity	Enlarged music sheet, sorting materials, picture book
Toileting	Long-handled cleaner, raised toilet seat with attached rails, bidet
Continence	Adult diaper, plastic liner
Bathing self	Grab bar, tub rail, bath seat, handheld shower hose, non-skid strips

---

ventions *continued* to be effective at the follow-up for 17 of these 19 problems (or 89% of the initially effective). As can be seen in Table 1, interventions were most successful for certain problems. These included the ADLs of feeding self, continence care, and bathing self, as well as the problems of engaging in behavior potentially dangerous to self, using stairs, and losing/misplacing things. The interviews with the caregivers indicated that, if introduced in

Table 1

Effectiveness of Project Interventions at Follow-up

Problem	Frequency	Effectiveness		Never Effective
		Initially Effective		
		Continued	No Longer	
Behavior dangerous to self	1	1		
Using stairs	1	1		
Forgetting the day	2		2	
Getting lost outside	2			2
Losing/misplacing things	2	2		
Feeding self	2	2		
Inactivity	3	1		2
Toileting	3			3
Continence	3	2		1
Bathing Self	10	8		2
Total	29	17	2	10

an appropriate manner by the caregiver and at a point in the disease when the patient was capable of making the necessary adjustments, the interventions for these problems tended to become incorporated into the daily behaviors and routines of the person with Alzheimer's disease and their caregivers. For only two of the problems (or 11%), however, were interventions initially but *no longer* effective at the follow-up. Both of these instances involved forgetting what day it was. While the intervention (a reality orientation board) was reported to have been appropriate for the person's initial level of cognitive functioning, it became ineffective as cognitive functioning declined.

On the other hand, interventions were deemed by the caregivers as having *never* been effective for 10 of the 29 problems addressed (or 34% of the total). It can be seen in Table 1 that interventions were least successful for the ADL of toileting, as well as the problems of getting lost outside the home and long periods of inactivity. For the problem of getting lost outside the home, there were specific explanations for intervention ineffectiveness: the identification bracelet was of the wrong length in one case, and was promptly destroyed by the patient in the other. Such clear explanations were absent, however, for the ineffectiveness of interventions for the problem of inactivity. Although all interventions took into account the person's past interests/hobbies, vocation, and current level of functioning, the reasons as to whether or not they actually became involved with a given intervention were unclear. Finally, the explanations for the ineffectiveness of interventions designed to assist with toileting were highly diverse. In one case, the intervention (a raised toilet seat with attached rails) was not made available because, although it may have assisted the person with Alzheimer's disease, it was difficult for the caregiver to use. In another case, the ineffectiveness of the intervention (a long-handled cleaner) appeared to have been due, at least in part, to the caregiver's lack of knowledge of how to introduce the intervention to their relative. In the third case, the ineffectiveness of the intervention (a bidet) appeared to have been due to either the caregiver's improper introduction of it to their relative, the strangeness of the object to the client and/or the caregiver's own observation that it was introduced too late in the course of the disease for the person to adapt to it.

DISCUSSION

The evaluation of the pilot project is instructive and encouraging. It suggests that professional assessment of the person with Alzheimer's disease and caregiver needs can pinpoint problems and expand the repertoire of solutions beyond those that caregivers can identify on their own. It is also evident that even with careful professional assessment and caregiver input in the selection of specific interventions for implementation, some interventions may be ineffective from the very outset. The reasons for intervention ineffectiveness, and their implications for minimizing such ineffectiveness are instructive in planning future programs.

First, caregivers may not be introducing interventions in an appropriate manner. Techniques which are gradual, persistent, and do not provoke negative reactions from the person with Alzheimer's disease may need to be taught to the caregiver. This suggests the importance of training by professionals when presenting caregivers with interventions. Second, because of caregiver preference, the interventions may not represent optimal choices for the person with Alzheimer's disease. In other words, the effectiveness of interventions may be problematic because, in some instances, what appears to be best for their relative is not necessarily best for the caregiver. Open discussions with the caregiver regarding expectations and priorities may shed light on such conflicts, and counseling of the caregiver may be warranted in some cases. Third, interventions may be introduced at a point in the disease when it is difficult, if not impossible, for the person with the disease to accept the change brought about by the intervention. In some cases, if the interventions are introduced while the person is still capable of acquiring new patterns of behavior, the interventions stand a much better chance of being effective.

At the same time, the finding that interventions which were initially effective still worked a number of months later for a very high percentage of problems is encouraging, especially in view of the progressive cognitive, physical, and behavioral decline which is a signature of Alzheimer's disease. These results suggest that progressive declines do not necessarily mean that interventions designed to assist caregivers are short-lived. On the contrary, some interventions can have relatively sustained impact if they can be implemented early. Attention to the needs of the person with the disease, caregiver preferences, caregiver skills, and timing in the course of the disease are all critical in establishing and maintaining the effectiveness of interventions.

CONCLUSIONS

The evaluation of the pilot research project suggests that problem identification and environmental interventions represent a promising approach in making caregiving for persons with Alzheimer's disease easier and safer. It is important to acknowledge that the findings reported are from a project with a small number of persons with Alzheimer's disease and their caregivers and addressed a particular set of problems with a specific set of caregiver-selected interventions. By the time of the follow-up, the project lost some of its most difficult cases to hospitalization or institutionalization. As a next step it would be useful to conduct such research with a larger number of participants and include other specific problems such as wandering or falling. In addition, it would be valuable to document, with the appropriate scientific rigor including controls, the manner in which interventions for such problems impact the stresses and capabilities of Alzheimer's disease caregivers.

REFERENCES

Alzheimer's Disease and Related Disorders Association. (1985). *Understanding and caring for the person with Alzheimer's disease*. Atlanta: Atlanta Area ADRDA Chapter.

Kern, T. (1986). Safety first: Modifying and adapting the environment for the patient with Alzheimer's disease. *Gerontology Special Interest Section Newsletter for Occupational Therapy, 9*, 4.

Pynoos, J., and Cohen, E. (1989). Environmental coping strategies for Alzheimer's caregivers. *The American Journal of Alzheimer's Care and Related Disorders & Research*, 4-8.

Pynoos, J., Cohen, E., and Lucas, C. (1988). *The Caring Home Booklet: Environmental Coping Strategies for Alzheimer's Caregivers*.

Pynoos, J. and Ohta, R. (1988). "Creating Better Environments for Alzheimer's Victims." Paper presented at the Annual American Society on Aging Conference, San Diego, California, March, 1988.

Skolaski-Pellitteri, T. (1984). Environmental intervention for the demented person. *Physical & Occupational Therapy in Geriatrics, 3*, 55-59.

Zarit, J.M. (1982). *Predictors of burden and distress for caregivers of senile dementia patients*. Unpublished doctoral dissertation, University of Southern California, Los Angeles.

Zarit, S.H., Reever, K.E., & Bach-Peterson, J. (1980). Relatives of the impaired elderly: Correlates of feelings of burden. *The Gerontologist, 20*, 649-655.

Zgola, J. (1990). Alzheimer's disease and the home: Issues in environmental design. *The American Journal of Alzheimer's Care and Related Disorders & Research*, 5-3.

Approaches to Problem Behaviors in Dementia

Margot Leverett, OTS

SUMMARY. Behaviors associated with dementia present serious management problems for nursing home staff and families of people with dementia. Sensory loss often compounds problems associated with dementia. This paper compares interventions focused on interaction and environment to those based on the medical model. Creating a closed unit for dementia patients is shown to be an effective way to provide care to people whose behavior is disruptive in other settings. In this study, use of an amplification device appeared to increase responsiveness and reduce the yelling behavior of an elderly woman with dementia and hearing loss.

Behaviors secondary to dementia present serious problems for families, nursing home staff and the patients themselves. These problem behaviors include wandering, combativeness and yelling. Wandering is a serious problem because it can result in the injury or death of the confused wanderer (Rader, 1987). Behaviors such as yelling and combativeness are upsetting and sometimes injurious to family members, staff, and other residents in a facility (McGrowder-Lin & Bhatt, 1988). Other problem behaviors include inappropriate removal of clothing, taking peers' belongings, frequent requests to be toileted without pathology, refusal to bathe, and banging on tables and chairs (McGrowder-Lin & Bhatt, 1988).

Margot Leverett is a graduate student in the Department of Occupational Therapy, University of Puget Sound, 1500 N. Warner, Tacoma, WA 98416.

The author wishes to thank Ron Stone, Kay Brittingham, Carol Nicholson, Steve Morelan, Joanne Rader, and audiologist Donnie Crowley for their valuable advice and assistance. Special thanks are extended to Louise Hall, Jacqueline Jewell, and Mary Rusdall for their assistance and cooperation throughout the project.

93

These behaviors have been called "excess disability," implying that they respond to treatment and are not an inevitable result of the disease process (Schwab, Rader & Doan, 1985). For the purposes of this paper, problem behaviors are defined as those behaviors that result in management problems or compromise the safety and comfort of the patient, including wandering, combativeness and yelling.

There are many theories about what causes problem behaviors, and a number of approaches to reducing them have been tried. The medical model focuses on elimination of a disease process through intervention directed at causal factors (Mosey, 1974). This study suggests that other models may be more appropriate for dealing with the sequelae of dementia. A comparison of approaches is illustrated in a case example.

REVIEW OF THE LITERATURE

A great deal of practical advice is available to caregivers of people with dementia (Griffin & Matthews, 1986; Gwyther, 1985; Macdonald, 1986; Mace, 1987; Rabins & Mace, 1981). However, few of the suggestions are supported by formal research. The literature on occupational therapy intervention for individuals with dementia has stressed the importance of assessment and activity analysis (Davis, 1986; Griffin & Matthews, 1986; Macdonald, 1986; Mace, 1985). Mace (1987) identifies general guidelines for selecting activities for dementia patients.

Causes of Problem Behaviors

There are various theories about the causes of problem behaviors of people with dementia. Bartol (1979) suggests that many of the behavior problems associated with dementia result from communication deficits. She recommends instructing staff in nonverbal communication techniques.

Sensory deprivation (Coons & Weaverdyck, 1986) and unskillful caregiver-patient interactions (Rader, Doan & Schwab, 1985; Rader, 1987) are cited as environmental factors contributing to problem behaviors. Hearing and other sensory loss can compound many problems associated with aging and disease (Falconer, 1986; Maloney, 1987). A pilot study by Maloney and Daily (1986) suggested that sensory stimulation may prevent further cognitive decline in patients with both sensory and cognitive losses.

Schwab and others (1985) suggest that problem behaviors are caused by anxiety arising from self-awareness of cognitive deficit. In another study by the same authors (Rader et al., 1985), it is suggested that people with dementia experience fear and loneliness caused by separation from the people and places with which they were previously most connected and comfortable. The steps an individual takes to relieve these feelings are referred to as agenda behavior.

Many authors concur that there is meaning in the confused behavior of people with dementia (Rader et al., 1985; Rader, 1987; Schwab et al., 1985; Schomaker, 1987). According to Rader (1987), people who wander are often attempting to return to a home or workplace that no longer exists. It is suggested that these people are trying to return to a state of mind rather than to a physical place.

In a study of retrospection by families of people with dementia (Schomaker, 1987), it was found that many apparently unintelligible behaviors were in fact perpetuations of previous, well-established behaviors that had been altered by the disease process. According to this study, the Alzheimer's disease process causes fragmentation, intensification, and increased frequency of many old behaviors, creating the illusion of a new behavior.

Approaches to Problem Behaviors

A number of approaches to problem behavior in people with dementia have been implemented. Bartol (1979) describes nonverbal communication techniques for use with dementia patients. The effectiveness of the techniques is documented in five case examples.

Work therapy has been used effectively with dementia patients. Griffin and Mouheb (1987) selected laundry folding as an activity for dementia patients who had been homemakers, because this activity was familiar to them. The authors stress the importance of basing activity selection on patients' past experience and providing a balance of work and leisure pursuits. Success of the laundry folding activity was documented in two case studies.

Comprehensive approaches have been successfully implemented at some facilities (Coons & Weaverdyck, 1986; Rader, 1987). These approaches employed a wide variety of valuable treatment techniques, from communication training to activities therapy. Reduced stimulation was combined with communication training and a structured activity program in a retirement residence (Cleary, Clamon, Price & Shullaw, 1988). Functional assessments, nursing reports and interviews indicated mixed results.

Sensory stimulation and exercise have been used in group formats with dementia patients (Maloney & Daily, 1986; McGrowder-Lin & Bhatt, 1988; Rader, 1987; Schwab et al., 1985). These programs required a high staff-patient ratio and involved a limited number of residents at a time. However, questionnaires, staff reports and assessments indicated functional improvements and reductions in problem behaviors in many residents who participated.

Many of the approaches to problem behaviors have proven too expensive or impractical for use in most care settings. Exercise and sensory stimulation programs are labor intensive and require special training of staff. Environmental approaches such as disguising exits or installing alarm systems to respond to exit-seeking wandering behavior are usually prohibitively expensive. The goal of this project was to find an approach to problem behavior that would be simple, versatile, and inexpensive enough to be used in a wide variety of settings.

Research for this project included observations of a closed Alzheimer's unit in a skilled nursing facility in Washington State. This discrete unit is reserved for residents with dementia and similar diagnoses. Residents who approach the single exit with intent to wander out are gently redirected, and are free to wander in the long hallway between the dining room and day room. Simply by setting aside one wing of a facility for demented residents, an environment is created in which unconventional behavior becomes the norm. No one is alarmed or annoyed when a resident who spends her days polishing the furniture polishes a few residents as well.

In a mixed unit, behaviors such as this can be very annoying to non-demented residents. Their expressions of annoyance, in turn, increase the demented person's self-awareness of deficit, which according to Schwab and others (1985), contributes to anxiety and results in more problem behaviors. This cycle is broken by creating a separate unit for residents with dementia.

METHOD

Problem behaviors are difficult to measure exactly. Wandering and combativeness are particularly difficult to quantify. Most of the studies presented here relied on reports of nursing staff for information about problem behaviors.

The original intent of this study was to measure the yelling behavior of an individual with dementia during one-hour periods once a day, and provide intervention intended to reduce agitation. Yelling was not measured during family visits or procedures such as bathing and dressing because it was believed that these situations would skew the data. However, observation revealed that it was during visits and procedures that the subject yelled most. This is what made the yelling a problem for staff and family. Baseline data showed very little yelling, but yelling continued to be a problem. Data collected in this way did not provide useful information about the problem. Consequently, the single subject format was abandoned and a decision was made to rely on staff reports and interviews.

The original format of this study also included an intervention based on the volition subsystem of the Model of Human Occupation (Kielhofner, 1985). In this subsystem, three ways in which activities acquire meaning to an individual are described. Meaning arises from the usefulness of activities to the social milieu (helping others or supporting a family); from the states that the activity evokes (calmness or excitement); or by association with past life situations (nostalgia).

It was believed that activities which appear to be useful to others, or evoke a feeling of serenity, or remind a person of something they enjoyed doing when their children were small, could help someone with dementia to feel more calm and at home in their present environment, and result in a reduction of problem behaviors. Application of an occupational frame of reference such as the Model of Human Occupation could provide a framework for finding activities that address the needs of individual patients. Looking at factors such as temporal orientation, pattern of interests, and present and past roles could help the therapist identify activities that would provide the patient with a sense of meaning and connectedness with the environment. Such activities could reduce the patient's loneliness and anxiety and result in fewer problem behaviors. This approach may be useful in treating clients in early stages of the disease. A similar approach was used successfully by Griffin and Mouheb (1987) in a work therapy program.

The subject of the present study, however, no longer appeared to recognize most members of her family, nor did she respond to objects and activities adapted from her past experience. The subject had been an accomplished pianist and loved cats. However, bringing stuffed toy cats and music activities into her environment failed to reduce her yelling behavior or produce any response at all.

Stuffed toy cats may have lacked the qualities that make experiences with real cats meaningful to people who love cats. Listening to music does not have the same meaning that playing music has. A different choice of objects and activities might have produced different results. It is also possible that the objects and activities selected were not adapted adequately to the subject's level of function. Further study might reveal ways of identifying or adapting objects at a more basic level. In this study, a decision was made to shift from the occupational frame of reference to a more rehabilitative or environmental approach.

Many studies have attempted to reduce problem behaviors by addressing presumed underlying causes such as anxiety (Cleary et al., 1988; McGrowder-Lin et al., 1988; Rader, 1987; Schwab et al., 1985). This approach fits the medical model which, according to Mosey (1974), focuses on elimination of a disease process through intervention directed toward causal factors or pathology. The cause of psychosocial dysfunction is often unknown, and its symptoms and sequelae are highly variable. Consequently Mosey states that the medical model is of limited usefulness in approaching psychosocial dysfunction. What this suggests for therapists is that approaching problem behaviors by focusing on presumed causal factors may be inadequate.

Mosey proposes the biopsychosocial model as an alternative to the medical model. The biopsychosocial model is oriented to the individual as he or she exists in a group of meaningful others, the "client-in-community." The major assumption of this model is that an individual has the right not only to be free of disease but to participate in the life of the community. The model provides occupational therapists with a theoretical framework for treating not just disease and its sequelae, but the individual in his or her social environment. Alzheimer's disease, which has been called a "caregivers' disease," may best be approached from this framework.

CASE STUDY

Mrs. J, a 78-year-old woman with primary degenerative dementia of the Alzheimer's type, was admitted to the closed Alzheimer's unit in a skilled nursing facility in 1987. Mrs. J had been an accomplished pianist and continued to play until about a year after admission.

Partial hearing loss was documented prior to admission but had not been assessed since. Mrs. J had used hearing aids. However, as her cognitive impairment progressed, she was no longer able to use the volume control effectively and she would consistently pull her hearing aids out of her ears. By the time of intervention in 1990, Mrs. J was consistently rejecting her hearing aids.

Mrs. J was receiving daily doses of pain medications for arthritis and a thyroid supplement. She was also being treated with anti-anxiety drugs and major tranquilizers in an attempt to control her disruptive behavior.

Mrs. J ambulated with assistance and was dependent in self care. Although she would sometimes make eye contact and speak, her responses tended to be inappropriate. She recognized her husband but did not appear to recognize her daughter.

Staff identified Mrs. J's episodes of loud incoherent yelling as disruptive and annoying to staff, residents and visitors. Staff observed that she tended to yell during procedures such as weighing, dressing and changing and during family visits, and that once she started yelling, she would sometimes continue for hours. It was impossible to involve her in group activities because her yelling was too disruptive to the other residents. Consequently Mrs. J spent most of her time alone in her room.

Observation revealed that the problem was not one of frequency but of intensity—Mrs. J did not yell often or all day, but she tended to yell when people were interacting with her, making these interactions uncomfortable for everyone in the unit.

The relation between yelling and agitation could not be clearly established. Her family believed that she yelled because she was trying to communicate and could not hear herself. At times, especially when her husband left or when staff was bathing her, the yelling was accompanied by a furrowing of the brow, turning the head to one side, and straining forward in the chair. At other times, it was not clear that Mrs. J was uncomfortable or unhappy while yelling. The yelling was for the most part incoherent, but occasionally a recognizable phrase emerged, such as "that's beautiful." Although the yelling was clearly a problem for those around her, it was not possible to determine whether yelling was a problem for Mrs. J.

Proceeding on the hypothesis that the yelling was related to hearing loss, an audiologist was consulted. Hearing loss was not re-evaluated at this point, but the audiologist suggested trial use of an amplification device called a Pocketalker. Less intrusive than a hearing aid, the device resembles a Walkman or transistor radio. It is battery-operated, and has a pocket-size amplifier with volume control, a small microphone, and a simple earphone. The Pocketalker costs about $120, but other versions of the device are available for as little as $17. The unit coordinator, activities staff and family members were instructed in use of the device, and a Pocketalker was provided for a trial period of one month.

RESULTS

Mrs. J was first introduced to the device during a family visit. Her husband put the earpiece into Mrs. J's ear and spoke quietly into the microphone, saying "can you hear me?" Mrs. J turned to her husband, made eye contact and said, "Yes, I can hear, but I'm not going to play." Excited by this answer, her husband quickly asked her several other questions, to which she did not respond. But when she started to yell later, he again spoke quietly to her using the device, and she stopped yelling. On several subsequent occasions Mrs. J stopped yelling when spoken to quietly using the device. On other occasions, particularly when she was very agitated, it had no apparent effect.

After using the Pocketalker with Mrs. J, the activities assistant reported:

> When I spoke into the microphone, she woke up, turned to me with a sweet smile, and said 'yes' gently, without yelling. I knew I had made contact with her. I was very happy. I said I loved her, and she just looked at me and smiled. Before we got the Pocketalker, she would respond, but not appropriately. I was very frustrated. I tried puppets and van rides, but I only had sporadic successes. Now the successes are more frequent.

Although the effect of the device cannot be distinguished from the calming effect of the presence of another person, caregivers are now addressing Mrs. J in a quiet voice, whereas they used to shout to accommodate her hearing loss. This is considerably less disruptive to the unit, as well as being more comfortable for the caregivers.

Initially, Mrs. J could not use the amplification device independently because she tended to pull it out of her ear and take it apart, as she had done with the hearing aids. This problem was solved by replacing the earplug with lightweight headphones, which are available at the same price and are less intrusive, and by placing the amplifier outside her field of vision, where it does not attract her attention.

Staff are enthusiastic about the device and are now using it with many other residents. The activities department has purchased one, and other departments are also applying to do so. Staff members have expressed relief at not having to shout, and their interaction with hearing impaired and yelling residents appears to have increased. Residents who could not participate in group activities previously can now do so using the device. Staff feel encouraged about reducing yelling behaviors in many residents.

Mrs. J's husband chose not to continue using the device after a few trials. Since Mrs. J is still unable to communicate effectively much of the time due to dementia, he feels that the device is of limited usefulness. However, he had believed that she was deaf, and learning that she does have residual hearing has perhaps improved the quality of his interactions with her. He frequently talks quietly to her now even without the device.

The effect of the amplification device on Mrs. J's yelling cannot be objectively quantified. At times she stops yelling spontaneously, or seems to respond to quiet conversation even without the device. At other times, she seems to respond much better with the device. Overall, her responsiveness appears to have improved, and her yelling during caregiver and family interactions appears to have decreased since introduction of the device.

Auditory stimulation provided by the device may have contributed to the change in Mrs. J's behavior. The change in the tone of voice used by caregivers, from yelling to quiet talking, may also have influenced Mrs. J's yelling responses. And it is possible that the device allows her to hear herself better, so that she no longer needs to yell to hear her own voice.

What is significant is the response of the staff and family members to introduction of the device on the unit. The yelling problem is no longer viewed as intractable, and staff are enthusiastic about adding the device to their repertoire of approaches. Staff and family members have increased efforts to communicate with Mrs. J, and are addressing her in a calm and quiet voice, which is more comfortable for everyone in the unit.

In a one month follow-up interview, nursing staff reported that Mrs. J has been provided with her own amplification device at a cost of under $20 and is using it independently about half of every day. The expense of battery replacement is cited as preventing full time use of the device at this facility, although Medicaid pays for battery replacement in many states. Staff report that Mrs. J is yelling less, that she often responds lucidly, follows simple verbal instructions, and stops yelling when asked using the amplification device. Nursing staff also report that Mrs. J has been taken off major tranquilizers and is doing better generally.

DISCUSSION

This study supports previous literature (Falconer, 1986; Maloney, 1987; Maloney & Daily, 1986) suggesting that sensory loss can compound problems associated with aging and dementia. When dealing with yelling behavior as a sequela of dementia, sensory loss may not be fully considered. Audiologists and other sensory specialists are valuable resources for the occupational therapist.

Observation of a closed Alzheimer's unit suggested that the unit itself solves many problems of behavior in dementia. The pounding on furniture, yelling, attempts to leave, and attempts to rearrange objects in the environment including other persons were all in evidence on the unit. However, as one family member pointed out, "of course these behaviors are a problem if the person is living at home. But on an Alzheimer's unit, where a person is surrounded with other people like himself or herself, the behavior is normal." Many behaviors that would make family or home life impossible are accepted without difficulty on the Alzheimer's unit. In that safe, protected and accepting environment, the behaviors remain, but the problems disappear. This supports the idea that problem behaviors are best approached in the social sphere.

One who investigates problem behaviors would do well to ask, "whose problem is it?" Although at times Mrs. J showed other signs of agitation and discomfort while yelling, the relation between yelling and discomfort could not be clearly established. Mrs. J could not tell us why she yelled or how it felt. It could not be determined whether the yelling was a problem for her.

There may be times when yelling has more meaning for Mrs. J than any of the activities staff try to engage her in. When all attempts to quiet Mrs. J fail after her husband leaves the facility to go home, it might not be appropriate to ask her to be calm. Yelling can be a meaningful response to a painful and unremediable situation. The "problem," if there is any, is in a cultural standard we have for adult behavior.

The difficulties in determining the cause of the yelling and the locus of the problem highlight Mosey's contention that the medical model is inadequate for dealing with the sequelae of psychosocial disabilities. In this case study, attempts to suggest causes of the yelling (agitation) and formulate treatment addressing the presumed cause (calming activities) failed or succeeded only intermittently. The most successful interventions involved restructuring the environment by creating an Alzheimer's unit and providing an amplification device.

The problem of yelling is in the social sphere. Consequently, the focus of intervention must be in the social sphere. In cases of psychosocial disability such as Alzheimer's disease, treatment directed at the individual according to the medical model will be less effective than treatment directed at the environment. It is possible to create environments where wandering is safe, pounding on the furniture is harmless, and yelling is a healthy expression of frustration. Problems can be solved even when behaviors can't be changed.

SUMMARY

The subject did not respond to attempts to reduce yelling behavior by introducing adaptations of objects and activities that had been meaningful to her in the past. It was suggested that a different choice of objects and more sensitive adaptations might produce better results. The occupational frame of reference may be more suitable for patients in earlier stages of the disease.

Use of an amplification device increased responsiveness of the subject and appeared to reduce the subject's yelling behavior. Staff responded enthusiastically to the device and reported increased interaction with hearing impaired residents. Literature suggesting that sensory loss compounds problems of dementia is substantiated by this study.

Many problem behaviors tend to be more problematic for caregivers than for the individual with dementia. The Alzheimer's unit appears to be an economical and effective way to provide safe, accepting and loving care to people whose behavior is disruptive in other settings. Future research could assess the impact of this type of care on people with dementia and their families.

REFERENCES

Bartol, M. A. (1979). Nonverbal Communication in Patients with Alzheimer's Disease. *Journal of American Nursing*, 5(4), 21-31.

Coons, D. H., & Weaverdyck, S. E. (1986). Wesley Hall: A Residential Unit for Persons with Alzheimer's Disease and Related Disorders. *Physical & Occupational Therapy in Geriatrics*, 4(3), 29-53.

Cleary, T. A., Clamon, C., Price, M., & Shullaw, G. (1988). A Reduced Stimulation Unit: Effects on Patients with Alzheimer's Disease and Related Disorders. *The Gerontologist*, 28(4), 511-514.

Davis, C. (1986). The Role of the Physical and Occupational Therapist in Caring for the Victims of Alzheimer's Disease. *Physical & Occupational Therapy in Geriatrics*, 4(3), 15-23.

Falconer, J. (1986). Aging and Hearing. *Physical & Occupational Therapy in Geriatrics*, 4(2), 3-19.

Griffin, R. M., & Matthews, M. U. (1986). The Selection of Activities: a Dual Responsibility. *Physical & Occupational Therapy in Geriatrics*, 4(3), 106-112.

Griffin, R. M., & Mouheb, F. (1987). Work Therapy as a Treatment Modality for the Patient with Dementia. *Physical & Occupational Therapy in Geriatrics*, 5(4), 67-72.

Gwyther, L. P. (1985). *Care of Alzheimer's Patients: A Manual for Nursing Home Staff*, American Health Care Association and Alzheimer's Disease and Related Disorders Association.

Kielhofner, G. (1985). *A Model of Human Occupation*. Williams and Wilkins.

Macdonald, K. C. (1986). Occupational Therapy Approaches to Treatment of Dementia Patients. *Physical & Occupational Therapy in Geriatrics*, 4(2), 61-72.

Mace, N. (1985). Home and Community Services for Alzheimer's Disease. *Physical & Occupational Therapy in Geriatrics*, 4(3), 5-14.

Mace, N. (1987). Principles of Activities for Persons with Dementia. *Physical & Occupational Therapy in Geriatrics*, 5(3), 13-28.

Maloney, C. C. (1987). Identifying and Treating the Client with Sensory Loss. *Physical & Occupational Therapy in Geriatrics*, 5(4), 31-45.

Maloney, C. C. & Daily, T. (1986). An Eclectic Group Program for Nursing Home Residents with Dementia. *Physical & Occupational Therapy in Geriatrics*, 4(3), 55-80.

McGrowder-Lin, R., & Bhatt, A. (1988). A Wanderer's Lounge Program for Nursing Home Residents with Alzheimer's Disease. *The Gerontologist*, 28(5), 607-609.

Mosey, A. C. (1974). An Alternative: the Biopsychosocial Model. *The American Journal of Occupational Therapy*, 28(3), 137-140.

Rabins, P. & Mace, N. L. (1981). *The 36-Hour Day*. Baltimore, MD: Johns Hopkins Press.

Rader, J. (1987). A Comprehensive Staff Approach to Problem Wandering. *The Gerontologist*, 27(6), 756-760.

Rader, J., Doan, J., & Schwab, M. (1985). How to Decrease Wandering, a Form of Agenda Behavior. *Geriatric Nursing*, July/August, 196-199.

Schwab, M., Rader, J., & Doan, J. (1985). Relieving the Anxiety and Fear in Dementia. *Journal of Gerontological Nursing*, 11(5), 8-15.

Schomaker, D. (1987). Problematic Behavior and the Alzheimer Patient: Retrospection as a Method of Understanding and Counseling. *The Gerontologist*, 27(3), 370-374.

Snyder, L., Rupperecht, P., Pyrek, J., & Moss, T. (1978). Wandering. *The Gerontologist*, 18(2), 272.

Conflicts in Managing Elderly Clients and Elderly Parents: The Dual Role of Health Professionals

Joanne M. Routzahn, MS, RN, CS

SUMMARY. Many nurses and other health professionals who are caring for aging parents also provide professional services to the elderly. This dual role of personal and professional caregiving is emotionally draining and influences clinical practice. This article identifies the feelings associated with caregiving, how these feelings influence professional practice and suggests strategies in coping with personal issues in family and professional settings.

Many nurses and other health professionals who are caring for aging parents also provide professional services to an aging population. Balancing personal and professional caregiving and processing the feelings associated with caregiving is difficult and emotionally draining as one superimposes one's own fear of aging, being alone, dependent on others and in poor health in later years. This dual role and triple-edged stress permeates the caregiving process affecting judgement and decision-making in professional practice. This article identifies the feelings associated with caregiving, how these feelings influence professional practice and suggests strategies in coping with personal issues in family and professional settings.

Joanne M. Routzahn is a certified Gerontological Nurse Specialist with over 25 years of nursing experience in community-based programs. She is a clinician, consultant and co-leader of support groups for caregivers of aging relatives and adult children of aging parents for Contra Costa County Geriatric Services. Address correspondence to the author at 2923 Macdonald Avenue, Richmond, CA 94804.

107

REVIEW OF THE LITERATURE

Caregiving is a multi-dimensional task (Clark et al., 1983). The literature has focused on understanding and coping with personal caregiving of families, namely spouses and adult children (Brody, 1985; Pruchno & Resh, 1989) with their feelings of burden, anger, guilt and anxiety (Baillie, 1987; Phillips, 1989) and strategies for coping (Mace & Rabins, 1981). The feelings associated with caregiving often produce caregiver stress. Studies have shown caregiver stress interferes with job performance (Travelers, 1985). The prevalence and extent to which caregiver stress and personal caregiving affect health professionals who are caring for aging clients have not been studied. Katz and Genevay (1987) have addressed how these feelings influence clinical practice when working with older clients but do not explore the dilemmas, concerns and needs of professionals having a dual role.

FEELINGS AND UNRESOLVED CONFLICTS INFLUENCING PROFESSIONAL PRACTICE

The dual role of adult caregiver to aging parents and nurse in professional practice is not uncommon. The stress of the dual role is compounded when role conflict or role overload is present. Given a significant number of older persons rely on working adult children, many of whom are health professionals serving the elderly, the dilemmas, conflicts and needs of the professional must be addressed in both the family and work settings.

Nurses and other health professionals bring not only their knowledge but their personal self, beliefs and emotions into interactions with clients and their families. This personal-professional connection is an opportunity to exchange energy and information. The delivery of care is based on this exchange (Rogers, 1970). In the human experience feelings that are generated by this interaction can lead to positive personal and professional growth. These feelings can also lead to errors in judgement and practice, however, if the professional fails to recognize and/or process them appropriately.

Working with older adults generates feelings and unresolved conflicts in professionals, many of whom are adult children of aging parents. These feelings and unresolved conflicts described by Katz and Genevay (1987) are anger, denial, the need to be needed, the need to control, the fear of one's own aging, the fear of death and professional omnipotence.

Using Katz and Genevay's model, areas of clinical practice reflecting the feelings and unresolved conflicts of the professional are numerous and could negatively affect the client as follows: fostering dependency; avoiding or rejecting the client; misperceiving symptoms and needs involving treatment issues; making unilateral decisions without respecting the right to autonomy and control in later years.

In the professional setting a framework dealing with these issues must be addressed when working with older clients. Oftentimes the issues are present but unnoticed or ignored as the client or family is labeled as "difficult" by failing to meet the criteria of the program, achieving the stated goals or refusing service. Overlooked is an integral element of the professional-client interaction, the underlying feelings and emotions of the professional which influences the delivery of care.

STRATEGIES IN COPING WITH PERSONAL AND PROFESSIONAL CAREGIVING

Discussions, case conferences and clinical supervision provide an opportunity to explore client-professional interactions more closely in terms of referrals, perceived needs, interventions and the manner in which the care is delivered.

Personnel policies need to address employee-caregiver concerns with policies that are sensitive to caregiver needs such as the use of sick time or flex time to respond to family crises; the use of personal or telephone time to consult or arrange for services to an aging parent or disabled spouse. Advocacy is needed on local, state and federal levels for Family Leave Acts that provide leaves of absence to respond to family needs without jeopardizing one's employments or benefits.

Finally, there must be recognition that health professionals are reluctant to admit or reveal their fear and anxiety in areas where they have been deemed proficient. Adult children of aging parents who are health professionals need guidance and support for this multi-dimensional task. Counseling, individual therapy or group support is indicated when these feelings and unresolved conflicts interfere with clinical practice. Support groups for adult children of aging parents are available to discuss feelings of anger, frustration and guilt enabling the participant to develop healthier strategies in coping with caregiving. Counseling is offered regarding aging, family dynamics, overcoming communication barriers and caregiver stress. Community resources are explored to ease the burden of caregiving.

CASE STUDY

The following case study describes an experienced middle-aged professional nurse's response to her dual role as an adult child of an aging parent and a professional provider of services to the frail elderly in a community-based program.

"I love my mother and I love my job. But lately the task of balancing the two, caring for my own family and meeting my own needs has overwhelmed me. My work is suffering. I feel angry, guilty, alone and depressed."

My mother is a 74 year old woman who has become legally blind in the last year forcing her to give up driving her car, reading the newspaper and balancing her checkbook. She has narcolepsy and the residual effects of polio from childhood along with arthritis and a progressive deterioration of her cervical spine rendering her left arm useless and her right leg atrophied. In addition to her bouts of lethargy and catalepsy spells, she falls frequently. My mother is becoming more dependent on me as her pace slows and her activities become more planned than spontaneous. As she struggles with her disabilities her sense of aloneness and melancholia, which have been life long, are increasing.

As my mother and I age together, we are more accepting and supportive of each other. We both keenly feel the brevity of time left as we put to rest the alienation and hurts of the past. When I step back and get in touch with my mother's aging and declining health, I begin to feel the anger and helplessness that burdened me as a child. As a child I suffered the consequences of her poor health over which I had no control and dealt with my fear by suppressing my feelings.

Now as a daughter of an aging parent and a middle-aged professional I am more aware of a dual role of personal and professional caregiver and how the feelings and unresolved conflicts in my personal life are evoked when working with frail older clients.

For example, one of my clients, an anxious frail 86 year old woman frequently called my office with vague complaints mostly stemming from her loneliness and need for attention. On this particular day I brushed aside her calls but decided to visit later that day. Finding her dead on the floor later that afternoon in many ways was a relief after months of struggling to maintain her in the community without an adequate support system.

Since she seemed fairly healthy and adamant about staying in her home I supported Mrs. A's decision to remain there despite numerous crises centering around her ability to care for herself. There was enormous pressure on me from her neighbors and other service providers to "do something." When the cause of death was later confirmed as tuberculosis, I was shocked and felt professionally inadequate for not recognizing her failing condition and guilty for not responding to her call quickly.

During this period my mother was staying with me and deteriorating as well. Because of this my anxiety increased at work which I then transferred onto my clients. On my day off I arranged for a 95 year old client to be brought by ambulance to a hospital for an evaluation of her vague complaints. "Nothing is wrong with her," said the emergency room physician.

In order to cope with my anxiety I suppressed my feelings and used denial as a defense mechanism. Yet these two clients triggered my fears which influenced my professional response, assessment and clinical decisions. The first client triggered my fear and inability to face the crisis in my personal life; namely the perceived death of my mother. Consequently I minimized Mrs. A's concerns and delayed responding to her. Not having dealt with my fear and guilt the second client triggered my feelings of doubt about my professional skills to the extent I overreacted and misjudged her condition. My personal life and professional caregiving had become intwined.

CONCLUSION

Having lost the boundaries of self which often occurs in daughters caring for aging parents, the impact of denial, guilt and death had a direct affect on this professional's practice as her suppressed feelings went unrecognized. Dealing with her anger, fear and unmet needs in a support group for adult children of aging parents this nurse was able to resolve some of these issues which she later explored with her clinical supervisor.

This case history illustrates the dilemmas, concerns and needs of health professionals in the dual role of managing elderly clients and elderly parents. In order to safeguard professional practice and ease the burden of personal and professional caregiving, feelings and emotions of health professionals serving the elderly must be addressed in the clinical setting. Research, education and training are needed to determine how these feelings and unresolved conflicts influence professional practice. Frameworks then need to be developed to deal with these issues in the professional setting.

REFERENCES

Baillie, V., Norbeck, J. & Barnes, L. Stress, social support and psychological distress of family caregivers to the elderly. *Nursing Research*, 1988, 37(4), 217-222.

Brody, E.M. Women in the middle and family help to older people. *The Gerontologist*, 1985, 25(1), 471-480.

Brody, E.M. Parent care as a normative family stress. *The Gerontologist*, 1985, 25(1), 19-28.

Clark, N. & Rakowski, R. Family caregivers of older adults: skills improving helping. *The Gerontologist*, 1983 23(6), 637-642.

Enright, R. & Friss, L. Employed caregivers of brain impaired adults: an assessment of the dual role. A Final Report to the Gerontological Society of America, 1986.

Mace, N. & Rabins P. *The 36 Hour Day*. Baltimore, MD: Johns Hopkins Press, 1981.

Phillips, L. Elder-family caregiver relationships: determining appropriate nursing interventions. *Nursing Clinics of North America*, 1989, 24(3), 795-805.

Pruncho, R. & Resh, N. Husbands and wives as caregivers: antecedents of depression and burden. *The Gerontologist*, 1989, 29(2), 159-164.

Rogers, M. *An Introduction to the Theoretical Basis of Nursing*. Philadelphia: F.A. Davis Company, 1970.

Travelers employee caregiver survey. The Traveler, Hartford, CT, June 1985.

Measuring the Functional Performance of Nursing Home Patients with the Bay Area Functional Performance Evaluation

William C. Mann, PhD, OTR
Linda Small Russ, OTR

The purpose of this study was to examine the use of the Bay Area Functional Performance Evaluation (BaFPE) Task Oriented Assessment (TOA) in measuring the functional status of patients in skilled nursing facilities (Lang and Bloomer, 1987), and to discuss the role of functional assessment with this population. Developed to assess patients in psychiatric settings, the BaFPE-TOA requires that patients individually participate in five activities: Sorting Shells, Money Marketing, Home Drawing, Block Design, and Draw a Person. The development and theoretical principles that underlie the BaFPE are described by Houston, Williams, Bloomer, and Mann (1989).

REVIEW OF LITERATURE

For nursing home patients, measurement of functional status of patients and the underlying causes of functional skill deficits is necessary to develop effective treatment strategies. Nursing home pa-

William C. Mann is Associate Professor and Chair, SUNY/Buffalo, Department of Occupational Therapy.

Linda Small Russ is Post Professional Degree Graduate Student, SUNY/Buffalo, Department of Occupational Therapy.

The authors wish to thank the Administrators of the Deaconess Skilled Nursing Facility, Buffalo, New York, for their cooperation in providing access to patients, and to Mary Beth Bunker and Penny Gabler for their help with the organizational aspects of patient testing.

113

tient characteristics have changed considerably over the last several years. Patients are now more ill and have greater functional deficits. Stull and Vernon (1986) point to the increased need for "more complicated treatments including: IV medication and hyperalimentation regiment, naso and gastro feedings, sterile dressing changes, tracheotomy care, and in some instances renal dialysis." Given that almost all nursing home patients have functional skill deficits, the occupational therapist must determine extent and cause of these deficits.

Assessment of older persons, including those not in nursing homes, must take into consideration characteristics that have been identified through previous research. Reaction time (the interval of time between a stimulus and a person's response) increases each year past the age of 20, and the rate of increase is even greater past the age of 60 (Birren, 1964). Motivation also changes with age, and older persons are less likely to respond to a question or task unless they are sure they will have the correct response. Older persons therefore, on average, achieve poorer scores (Birkhill, 1975). Timed tests, and tests which contain items or tasks that do not have immediate relevance, may be less useful for older persons.

While there have been studies demonstrating the importance of activity and the relationship to functional status, self-concept, and perception of roles, measurement of functional status of nursing home patients has not been addressed recently in the occupational therapy literature. Studies by occupational therapists of elderly and institutionalized persons point out the importance of activity and functional independence. Aitken (1982) studied the relationship of functional independence to self-concept in the hospitalized elderly, and found that dependent older persons had a lower self-concept. Duellman, Barris, and Kielhofner (1986) found a relationship between amount of organized activities offered in nursing homes and patients' perceptions of their present and future roles. Smith, Kielhofner, and Watts (1986, p. 278) studied the relationship between life satisfaction and volition and activity patterns in the elderly and concluded: ". . . Occupational therapists may enhance the life satisfaction of their elderly patients by emphasizing interests, values, personal causation, work, and leisure in their treatment programs." In a study of the use of a life review activity with confused nursing home patients, Kiernat (1979, p. 306) determined that "behaviors of confused residents improved during group meetings and that participants who attended most frequently showed the greatest change in behavior."

Measurement of functional status of elderly persons has received some attention by other disciplines. In a study of non-institutionalized elderly, Ford et al. (1988) used a combination of interview and self report to measure functional status and concluded self report alone is not a reliable method. Herbert, Carrier and Bilodeau (1988) developed the Functional Autonomy Measurement System (SMAF). The SMAF is based on the World Health Organization's classification of disabilities, and includes activities of daily living, mobility, communication, and mental functions. Scales have been developed for assessing elderly persons in the community (Golden, Teresi, and Gurland, 1984; Fillenbaum, 1985). The BaFPE is unique among all measures reviewed in that it requires observation and scoring of patients while they perform five separate tasks. This observation of actual task performance, in a standardized format, suggested that the BaFPE might be very useful in providing reliable information on functional status.

METHODS

Forty-two patients were randomly selected from a 162 bed skilled nursing facility in Buffalo, New York. The facility is one unit of a not-for-profit private health care system that also includes a University at Buffalo Health Sciences Center affiliated hospital. The facility offers a full range of rehabilitation services. The Occupational Therapy Department includes two full time certified occupational therapy assistants (COTAs) and a part time (one day per week) occupational therapist (OTR).

The forty-two patients in this study ranged in age from 47 to 93 years old, with 85% of the patients 65 years old or older. Almost half of the sample were 80 years old or older. The mean age was 75.4 years, and the median was 79 years. The sample included thirteen men (31%) and twenty-nine women (69%). Total length of stay from first nursing home admission ranged from two months to four years, four months. Mean and median length of stay was one year, six months.

An OTR working toward a post professional MS degree in occupational therapy administered the BaFPE-TOA. This OTR was not an employee or consultant of the nursing home. Each patient was tested in a private testing room. Administration of the BaFPE-TOA took between 45 and 60 minutes for each patient.

The BaFPE-TOA includes five tasks that are rated on a five point scale: Sorting Shells (ten categories of shells are sorted by shape, size, and color); Money and Marketing (patients calculate the cost of items on a shopping list, cash a check, and calculate change); Home Drawing (patients draw a floor plan for a house, following specific instructions); Block Design (patients duplicate a block design from memory or with the use of a cue card); and Draw a Person (patients draw a picture of a person doing something).

The BaFPE-TOA provides summary scores for each of the five tasks, as well as scores for three Components: Cognitive, Performance, and Affective. Each component has sub-components or "Parameters." The evaluator uses a rating sheet with specific guidelines for scoring patients on twelve Parameters for each task. There is also a section called "Qualitative Signs and Referral Indicators" (QSRI) which allows the evaluator to check for general signs of an organic disorder that are observable during all five tasks. The QSRI score is obtained by rating patients on Language, Comprehension, Hemispatial Neglect, Memory, Abstraction, and Task Specific observations on each of the five tasks.

RESULTS

This section will present results for each of the five tasks, for the QSRI, and for the Component scores for the BaFPE-TOA.

Task Scores

Table 1 provides a summary of the results of patient performance on each of the five tasks. For Sorting Shells, seventeen percent of the patients in this study received the lowest possible score, while forty-seven percent scored at or below the midpoint of possible scores. (The lowest possible score is 12, the highest is 48, and the midpoint is 30, for all BaFPE-TOA tasks.)

On the Money Management task, twenty-six percent of the sample were rated at the lowest possible score, while eighty-six percent

TABLE 1: ANALYSIS OF TASK SCORES FOR BAPPE—TOA

TASK	% AT LOWEST SCORE	% OF PATIENTS ≤ 30	HIGHEST SCORE ACHIEVED	MEAN SCORE	MEDIAN SCORE	STANDARD DEVIATION
SORTING SHELLS	17%	47%	40	28	31	8.6
MONEY AND MARKETING	26%	86%	44	22	23	10.0
HOME DRAWING	29%	76%	44	21	20	11.5
BLOCK DESIGN	24%	57%	45	25	28	11.3
DRAW A PERSON	29%	64%	41	23	26	12

Lowest Possible Score = 12, Highest Possible Score = 48

117

scored at or below the midpoint score. Of all the BaFPE-TOA tasks, patients had the most difficulty with Money Management.

For the Home Drawing task, twenty-nine percent of the patients in this study could not do this task at all, while seventy-six percent scored at or below the midpoint score. One patient during this part of the testing became angry and stated: "I do not expect to buy a home." Another patient drew a plan that resembled a nursing home floor plan (Figure 1). Both patients were limited in ability to abstract.

On the Black Design Task, twenty-four percent of the patients received the lowest score, while fifty-seven percent scored at or below the midpoint score. On the Draw a Person task, twenty-nine percent of the patients in this study received the lowest possible score, while sixty-four percent scored at or below the midpoint score. Figure 2 provides some representative drawings for this task.

Qualitative Signs and Referral Indicators (QSRI)

Table 2 provides a summary of findings on the QSRI. For each task seventy-nine percent of the patients had at least one referral indicator. The mean number of indicators ranged from 4 to 5.8 across the five tasks. The highest number of indicators was 17, for Sorting Shells.

Component/Parameter Scores

Table 3 provides a summary of the Component/Parameter scores for the BaFPE-TOA. On the Cognitive Component, thirty percent of the patients received the lowest score. The mean score was 47.1 across a range of possible scores of 25 to 100. A closer examination of the Cognitive Component is provided in Table 4. For Memory for Written/Verbal Instruction, forty-eight percent of the patients received the lowest score, and the mean score was 6.9 in a possible score range of 5 to 20.

For Organization of Time and Materials, thirty-four percent of the patients received the lowest score. The mean score was 8.2 out of a range of possible scores from 5 to 20.

Scores for the Attention Span Parameter were low, but not as low as the Memory and Organization Parameters. Twenty-seven percent of the patients received the lowest score and the mean score was

FIGURE 1: EXAMPLE

OF HOME DRAWING

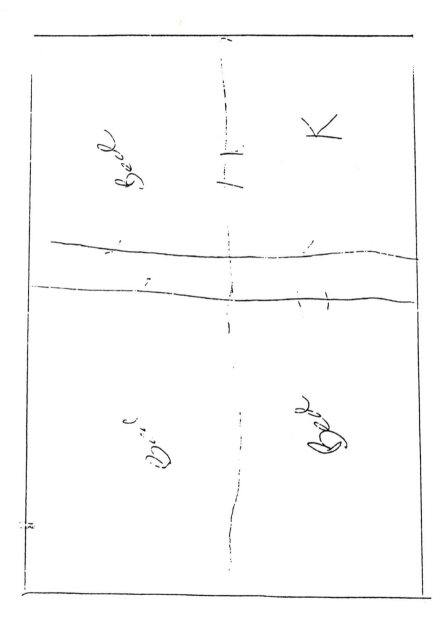

FIGURE 2 :

EXAMPLES OF DRAW A PERSON

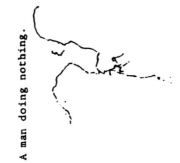

A man doing nothing.

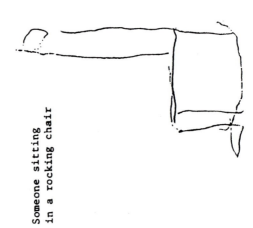

Someone sitting
in a rocking chair

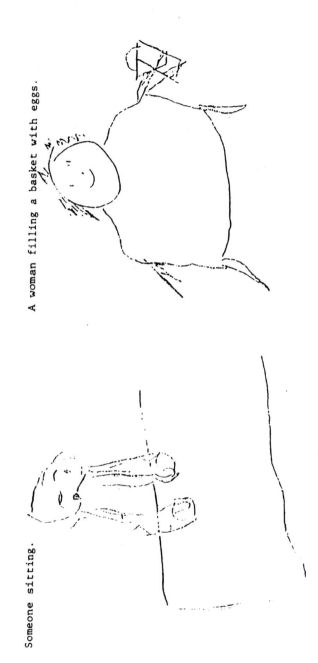

A woman filling a basket with eggs.

Someone sitting.

TABLE 2: ORGANICITY: ANALYSIS OF QUALITATIVE SIGNS & REFERRAL INDICATORS FOR BAPPE – TOA

TASK/MEASURE	% WITH AT LEAST ONE SIGN	MEAN	MEDIAN	STANDARD DEVIATION	HIGHEST NUMBER OF SIGNS
SORTING SHELLS	83%	5.8	5.0	4.3	17
MONEY AND MARKETING	83%	4.7	4.0	3.4	14
HOME DRAWING	81%	4.0	3.5	3.4	13
BLOCK DRAWING	79%	5.4	5.5	4.1	13
DRAW A PERSON	79%	4.9	4.0	4.3	13

TABLE 3: ANALYSIS OF COMPONENT/PARAMETER SCORES FOR BAFPE – TOA

	% AT LOWEST SCORE	MEAN	MEDIAN	STANDARD DEVIATION	HIGHEST SCORE
COGNITIVE*	30%	47.1	51	23.5	91
PERFORMANCE**	41%	18.5	19.5	8.9	37
AFFECTIVE***	25%	46.3	50	21.6	79

* Lowest Possible Score = 25, Highest Possible Score = 100

** Lowest Possible Score = 15, Highest Possible Score = 60

*** Lowest Possible Score = 20, Highest Possible Score = 80

123

TABLE 4: ANALYSIS OF COGNITIVE COMPONENT SCORES

	% AT LOWEST SCORE	MEAN	MEDIAN	STANDARD DEVIATION	HIGHEST SCORE
MEMORY FOR WRITTEN/VERBAL INSTRUCTION	48%	6.9	6.0	3.9	15
ORGANIZATION OF TIME AND MATERIALS	34%	8.2	8.0	4.2	18
ATTENTION SPAN	27%	10.7	11.0	5.5	20
EVIDENCE OF THOUGHT DISORDER	27%	12.8	13.5	6.8	20
ABILITY TO ABSTRACT	36%	8.4	9.5	5.1	18

Lowest Possible Score = 5, Highest Possible Score = 20

10.7. Similarly on the Evidence of Thought Disorder Parameter, twenty-seven percent of the patients received the lowest score, and the mean score was 12.8. Scores were lower on the Ability to Abstract Parameter, with 36 percent of patients receiving the lowest score, and the mean score was 8.4 in a range of possible scores from 5 to 20.

DISCUSSION

Task Scores

Visual impairments and decreased sensation account for some of the difficulty patients experienced with this task. The Sorting Shells task requires ability to separate items based on color, shape, and size. However, the greatest problem related to cognition, which will be discussed separately below. Of all five tasks, patients did relatively better on sorting shells, and seemed more comfortable in working on this task. Many occupational therapy programs in nursing homes use similar activities, although more often with pegs than with shells. Patients enjoy the environmental interaction afforded by this activity.

Patients had much more difficulty with the Money Management task than with the Shell Sorting Task. Most patients in nursing homes do little or no shopping, and may have forgotten how to manage money. The higher level cognitive processes involved in the calculations and problem solving represent another challenge. The highly dependent role of nursing home patient may be an important external factor in explaining the poor performance on this task. During trips outside the nursing home, it would be far more therapeutic to have patients handle their own money, with assistance as needed, than to have an activity director make a single payment for the group. Setting up shopping activities in the nursing home, and encouraging patients to participate would provide additional money management experiences. Practice shopping exercises with paper and pencil in occupational therapy, similar to this BaFPE task, could also help stimulate patient interest.

The Home Drawing task asks patients to draw a floor plan of a house. Many patients had difficulty with this. While cognitive limitations may account for some of this difficulty, there may also be a strong emotional component. Many patients have lost their homes and their loved ones they lived with in their home. Therapists using the BaFPE should consider this, and provide time for discussion after completing the BaFPE. In some sensitive cases it might be best to not use the BaFPE at all. Figure 1 presents a plan that resembled a nursing home floor plan, reflecting institutionalization.

The Block Design task requires patients to duplicate a block design by memory, or with the assistance of a cue card if needed. Of the five tasks, this one would be rated less difficult than all but the Sorting Shells task. Like Sorting Shells, this is similar to activities often used in nursing home occupational therapy programs.

The Draw a Person task requires the patient to draw a picture of a person doing something. It is interesting to note that with but a few exceptions, the drawings reflected very passive activities. As stated by the patients, these included: "a man looking around"; "someone sitting"; "a man in a rocking chair"; and "a man doing nothing." Of the few active drawings, the activities either reflected activities done in occupational therapy, or activities associated with an early period of life: "knitting a lap robe"; and "a woman filling a basket with eggs."

Qualitative Signs and Referral Indicators (QSRI)

The findings from the Qualitative Signs and Referral Indicators suggest a high degree of organicity among this population. While this may have been expected, often mental status is not directly addressed in occupational therapy treatment.

Component/Parameter Scores

Table 3 provides a summary of the Component/Parameter (CP) scores for the BaFPE-TOA. The Cognitive Component includes (1) Memory for Written/Verbal Instruction, (2) Organization of Time and Materials, (3) Attention Span, (4) Evidence of Thought Disorder, (5) Ability to Abstract. The Performance Component includes (1) Task Completion, (2) Errors, and (3) Efficiency. The Affective Component includes (1) Motivation or Compliance, (2) Frustration Tolerance, (3) Self-confidence, and (4) General Affective and Behavioral Impression. Patients scored low on the Cognitive Component. Clearly, there are many problems associated with cognition, and these impact on functional performance.

Patients scored very low on the Memory for Written/Verbal Instruction parameter. Memory impairment impacts on functional performance in general, and on test taking. A test such as the BaFPE, where instructions are given only during the testing may not truly indicate the potential of the person to learn, and to complete functional activities. Therapists working with this population know the importance of daily instruction and repetition in Activities of Daily Living training. A compensatory approach commonly used with persons with head injuries is to use memory aids such as posted notes. This might also help nursing home patients with memory deficits.

Organization of Time and Materials also shows low scores, although not as low as the Memory Parameter. Organization of Time and Materials is very important for task initiation. Many nursing home patients can complete tasks "with setup." Treatment plans should consider practice in organizing materials and time as an important area in maintaining and regaining functional independence.

Most nursing home patients have multiple diagnoses and a mix of physical, sensory, cognitive, and behavioral impairments. In this sample, one patient was aphasic, and several others had verbal impairments. One patient was very anxious and this anxiety interfered with her attending to tasks. Other patients had tremors. Many patients had visual or hearing impairments. A few patients were very lethargic—one fell asleep in the middle of the test. Of all problems though, cognitive impairments were most prevalent, and posed the greatest challenge in administering the BaFPE-TOA. Likewise, cognitive impairments challenge therapists in helping nursing home patients maintain or regain functional skills.

CONCLUSIONS AND RECOMMENDATIONS

While several patients were able to participate in the tasks required for the BaFPE-TOA, a majority of patients did not complete either some or all of the activities. The BaFPE-TOA is appropriate for nursing home patients at the middle and higher end of cognitive and physical abilities, but for some patients, as many as twenty-five percent, it is not practical. In some cases use of the BaFPE-TOA could be frustrating to patients who are aware of their inability to complete the tasks. An initial screening is suggested before administering the BaFPE-TOA.

Having considered functional assessment and explored the use of the BaFPE-TOA with nursing home patients, the authors offer the following recommendations that go beyond the use of the BaFPE, but are suggested on the basis of this study experience:

1. Therapists should address cognitive status in evaluation and treatment of nursing home patients with at least the same level of attention afforded physical status. Even simple activities like sorting pegs or shells provide stimulation.
2. Therapists and administrators must recognize the role of environmental stimulation on cognitive status. The more sterile the environment, and the less interaction patients have with other people and with the environment, the more quickly they are likely to suffer a decline in cognitive status.
3. Occupational therapists should consider increased use of drawing, followed by discussion, as a way to stimulate thought and memory.
4. Research is needed on the effectiveness of certain activities. The relative success with, and enjoyment of, shell sorting suggests a need to better understand the impact of this and similar activities on a patient's functional status. The drawings suggest a lifestyle that is lonely, with little or no meaningful activity, which also supports the need for additional research.
5. Further research on the BaFPE with this population should examine the relationship between BaFPE scores and activities of daily living status.

REFERENCES

Aitken, M.J., (1982). Self-concept and functional independence in the hospitalized elderly. *American Journal of Occupational Therapy*, 36(4), 243-250.
Birkhill, W.R., Schaie, K.W. (1975). The effect of differential reinforcement of cautiousness in intellectual performance among the elderly. *Journal of Gerontology*, 30:578.

Birron, J.E. (1964). *The Psychology of Aging*, Englewood Cliffs, NJ: Prentice-Hall.

Duellman, M.K., Barris, R., Kielhofner, G. (1986). Organized activity and the adaptive status of nursing home residents. *American Journal of Occupational Therapy*, 40(9), 618-622.

Fillenbaum, G.G. (1985). Screening the elderly. A brief instrumental activities of daily living measure. *Journal of the American Geriatrics Society*, 33(10), 698-706.

Ford, A.B., Folmar, S.J., Salmon, R.B., Medalie, J.H., Roy, A.W., Galazka, S.S. (1988). Health and function in the old and very old. *Journal of the American Geriatrics Society*, 36(3), 187-97.

Golden, R.R., Teresi, J.A., Gurland, B.J. (1984). Development of indicator scales for the Comprehensive Assessment and Referral Evaluation (CARE) interview schedule. *Journal of Gerontology*, 39(2), 138-46.

Hebert, R., Carrier, R., Bilodeau, A. (1988). The Functional Autonomy Measurement System (SMAF): description and validation of an instrument for the measurement of handicaps. *Age and Ageing*, 17(5), 293-302.

Houston, D., Williams, S.L., Bloomer, J., Mann, W.C. (1989). The Bay Area Functional Performance Evaluation: development and standardization. *American Journal of Occupational Therapy*, 43(3), 170-183.

Kiernat, J.M. (1979). The use of life review activity with confused nursing home residents. *American Journal of Occupational Therapy*, 33(5), 306-310.

Lang, S., Bloom, J. (1987). Bay Area Functional Performance Evaluation, Second Edition. Palo Alto, CA: Consulting Psychologists Press.

Smith, N.R., Kielhofner, G., Watts, J.H. (1986). The relationships between volition, activity pattern, and life satisfaction in the elderly. *American Journal of Occupational Therapy*, 40(4), 278-283.

Stull, M.K., Vernon, J. (1986). Nursing care needs are changing in facilities with rising patient acuity. *Journal of Gerontological Nursing*, 12, 15-19.

Effects of a Multi-Strategy Program Upon Elderly with Organic Brain Syndrome

Velma Russ Reichenbach, MAMS, OTR/L
Margaret M. Kirchman, PhD, OTR/L, FAOTA

SUMMARY. The differential effects of a Multi-strategy Group Program and that of traditional nursing home care upon elderly residents with organic brain syndrome were measured using the Mental Status Questionnaire, the Face-Hand Test, the Philadelphia Geriatric Morale Scale, and Lowenthal's Langley-Porter Physical Self Maintenance Scale. Seventy two subjects with organic brain syndrome were assessed on morale, physical self-maintenance, and mental function before and after receiving the Multi-strategy Program or traditional nursing home care. Subjects in the Multi-strategy Programs showed significant improvement in morale, activities of daily living, and mental functioning following four months of intervention, while the traditional nursing home care group showed significant decrease in the same areas.

INTRODUCTION

By the year 2000 severe dementias are expected to affect 2.3 million people with resulting human suffering and enormous financial burden (Hellmick, 1988). The prevalence of severe dementia among those 65 to 74 is about 1 percent compared with 25 percent for those over 84 years of age. Dementia is the major cause of

Velma Reichenbach is Manager of Occupational Therapy Services at Medical Personnel Pool, 1515 N. Harlem, Oak Park, IL 60302, and is Consultant to Long Term Care Facilities. This study was in partial fulfillment of a master's thesis. Margaret M. Kirchman, Emerita, University of Illinois at Chicago, chaired her thesis committee.

institutionalization of the elderly (Fabiszewiski et al., 1988). Nursing home costs are 41 billion per year for patients with Alzheimer's disease, which accounts for 66% of the dementias (Congressional Summary, 1987). Zarit (1986) reports that preliminary studies suggest 20 percent of nursing home patients are inappropriately diagnosed as demented. McPhee (in Bach et al., 1988) reports that five to forty percent of clinically diagnosed Alzheimer cases are verified as incorrect upon autopsy.

Organic brain syndrome, which encompasses all of the dementias, is not a disease but a complex of symptoms that is difficult to define and diagnose (Bondareff, 1986). It can be acute (reversible) or chronic (irreversible) (Bussee and Pfeiffer, 1977; Henry, 1986). If acute brain syndrome is not treated it can become chronic and irreversible (Eisdorfer and Cohen, 1978, Cohen and Eisdorfer 1985, Henry, 1986). For many years cerebrovascular problems were incorrectly regarded as the primary cause of chronic brain syndrome. Now it is felt that only 15 to 25 percent fall in this category (Cohen and Eisdorfer, 1985).

Therapists need to be aware of the developing knowledge related to dementias and the potential of misdiagnosis. Difficulty in diagnosis occurs because mental or cognitive impairment in the elderly is not one set of symptoms or causes, but is influenced by biological, sociological and psychological factors (Cohen and Eisdorfer, 1985). Diagnosing must be considered from the whole person point of view (Butler and Lewis, 1973; Ernst, 1978, Cohen and Eisdorfer, 1986, Henry, 1986). Cohen and Eisdorfer (1986) have identified several factors clinicians need to note in differentiating problems of organic brain syndrome: (1) A person with chronic brain syndrome may develop a superimposed acute syndrome, (2) Chronic brain syndrome may or may not be of acute onset; however, without treatment, permanent structural damage may occur, (3) Treatability should be distinguished from reversibility, (4) There is variability in the functional capacity of individuals with organic brain syndrome.

Organic brain syndrome is not necessarily the fixed condition it appears to be and treatment often is the only reliable way to judge its reversibility (Butler and Lewis, 1973, Ernst, 1978). Acute confusional states or co-existing psychiatric conditions may be superimposed over a chronic condition; proper programming can improve well-being, promote comfort and enhance quality of life (Fabiszewski et al., 1988).

There is increasing awareness of the need for programs to influence maximum level of functioning, preserve comfort and esteem. Kern (1988) stresses tertiary prevention for preventive practice in Alzheimer's disease and in all work with the elderly population.

PURPOSE OF STUDY

The purpose of this study was to examine the effects of Multi-strategy Group Programs and the effects of traditional nursing home care upon elderly residents diagnosed as having organic brain syndrome. It also was to compare the Multi-strategy Group Programs to traditional nursing home care and to determine if there was a difference in these two groups within three categories of organic brain syndrome: (1) mild, (2) moderate, and (3) severe.

There were three null hypotheses:

1. There is no difference in pre and post Multi-strategy Group Program measurements on morale, mental function, and activities of daily living for elderly nursing home residents within three categories of organic brain syndrome: (1) mild, (2) moderate and (3) severe, nor in all three groups combined.

2. There is no difference in pre and post measurements of morale, mental function and activities of daily living on residents receiving traditional nursing home care only, within three categories of organic brain syndrome; (1) mild, (2) moderate and (3) severe, nor in all three groups combined.

3. There is no difference between the effects of the Multi-strategy Group Program and the effects of traditional nursing home care on residents within three categories of organic brain syndrome: (1) mild, (2) moderate and (3) severe, nor in all groups combined.

METHODOLOGY

This study was conducted in two 100 bed licensed intermediate care nursing homes in the Chicago metropolitan area. Both facilities were attached to retirement villages. They were alike in having residents from their own facility within the nursing areas as well as elderly admitted from the community as nursing home patients. Permission for testing and carrying out the program was granted by the administration and house physicians of the facilities. Consent forms were secured.

Assessments Used in the Study

The scales selected for this study because of their brevity, validity and reliability were the Mental Status Questionnaire (Kahn and Goldfarb, 1960), the Face Hand Test (Bender, 1975, Fink, Green and Bender, 1952), the Philadelphia Geriatric Morale Scale (Lawton, 1972), and the Physical Self Maintenance Scale (Lawton and Brody, 1969).

The Mental Status Questionnaire and the Face Hand Test have been adapted for determining organic brain impairment. Kahn (1971) used them for a large survey comparing the population of three types of institutions: nursing homes, homes for the aged and state hospitals. For this study an adapted rating scale used scores of 0-3, 4-7, and 8-10 representing mild, moderate and severe dysfunction. The errors provide an index to severity and can be used to indicate change over time (Kahn and Miller, 1978).

Bender developed the Face-Hand Test in 1952 while studying disorders of perception. This test elicits defects in perception of simultaneous tactile stimuli in the aged. The older the subject the more likely the impairment. Defects increase in frequency and severity with increased mental dysfunction. This test has proven to be empirically effective providing a continuum of dysfunction as well as differentiating organic from non organic brain syndrome (Bender, 1975; Kahn and Miller, 1978).

The Philadelphia Geriatric Center Morale Scale (PCG) was developed by Lawton (1975). It was first used on elderly people both in institutionalized settings and in their own homes and is designed for normally responsive and marginally comprehending elderly subjects. A 17 item scale contains three separate and stable factors, agitation, attitude toward own aging, and lonely dissatisfaction. Two replication studies, one by Lawton (1975) and another by Morris and Sherwood (1975) demonstrated that a shortened, revised scale is stronger, and a more accurate measure than the original. Research demonstrated that the reliability values between the original and revised scales are very similar, and the interscale levels of correlation are extremely high. The revised scale was used in this study.

The Physical Self Maintenance Scale has been adapted from Lowenthal's Langley-Porter Physical Self-Maintenance Scale, by Lawton and Brody (1969). Independence in the self-care areas is scored as one, all other levels of dependence are scored as zero. In this study zero will indicate complete dependence and four will indicate complete independence in each area of daily living activities. This alternate method of scoring will not change the scale.

Selection of Subjects

Three steps were taken in selecting subjects. A review of the charts was done and those residents over the age of 65 with a diagnosis indicating organic brain syndrome were chosen as possible subjects. All of the subjects were described in the charts as having varying symptoms of organic brain disorder. Residents were required to have communication ability to answer simple questions. Seventy-two subjects were selected from the group of 100 residents identified with a diagnosis of organic brain syndrome. To make this selection, screening was done using the Face-Hand Test (Bender, 1952) and the Mental Status Questionnaire (Kahn et al., 1960, Goldfarb, 1974). These tests were administered to 45 and 47 respectively of the 50 subjects, in each facility. The testing of this many subjects was required to fill the quota of 12 mild, 12 moderate, and 12 severe organic brain syndrome subjects, resulting in 36 subjects in each facility. When administrating the Face-Hand Test, if a subject made a mistake on identifying where he/she had been touched simultaneously on the trials of 1-4, 5-8, or after 8, he/she was placed in the appropriate mild, moderate or severe category of Organic Brain Syndrome. A Random Numbers Table was used to place them in one of two groups; the Multi-strategy Group that received the therapeutic strategies, or the control group that received traditional nursing home care.

Assessing the Subjects

The four instruments previously described were used to assess all subjects in the areas of morale, mental function, and activities of daily living. To assess subjects, answers to questions on the Mental Status Questionnaire were obtained through conversation. The Morale questions were read to the subjects; and subjects were requested to think about the questions and respond with yes or no as to their true feelings. For the Face-Hand Test, subjects were told that a test of perception would be done, first with the eyes closed and then with the eyes open. (The subject was lightly touched simultaneously on one hand and one cheek.) A subject who would correctly answer where he/she had been touched after trial five or six was presumed free of brain damage. The activities of daily living scores were obtained from questioning the nurse or aide who worked most often with the resident. This was done by going over the statements in the Physical Self-Maintenance Scale with the nurse or aide and making sure there was no discrepancy in interpretation of the statements as the subject was scored. These methods of obtaining measurements were done for all subjects. Testing took place at similar times of the day, within a two week period prior to, and following a four month period of intervention for both the Multi-strategy Group and for the control group that received traditional nursing home care.

Occupational therapists familiar with the instruments performed the testing following a review of the procedures to assure similar testing approaches.

Multi-strategy Program

The leaders of the Multi-strategy program were activity aides with a high school education. They were chosen through consultation with the activity department supervisor. Good listening skills, an ability to relate and develop rapport with older persons, a genuine concern for the residents' well being, and a desire to learn about the aging process were required. Prior work as an activity worker provided them with some knowledge of reality orientation, reminiscence and remotivation techniques. The occupational therapist provided them with four hours of inservice related to myths of aging, psychosocial social theories and concepts such as the spiral of senility. Another four hours of weekly guidance was provided by the therapist during the intervention period.

One hour of inservice education was provided all facility staff, to familiarize them with the purpose of the program and to engage their support in assisting and encouraging the residents' attendance at the Multi-strategy Group Programs.

The Multi-strategy Program was intended to counteract the many deprivations that lead to insufficient stimulation, disorganized behavior, lowered self esteem, depression, and cortical inactivity that can cause multiple symptoms of organic brain syndrome (Oster, 1976; Parent, 1978; Frengley, 1987). Deprivation factors are illustrated in Reichenbach's (1981) diagram (Appendix A).

The program was held five mornings a week for one hour over a four month period. Reality orientation, remotivation, sensory stimulation and integration, reminiscence, and exercises were used with an underlying theme of esteem building.

Orientation took place in a subtle way, unlike the original reality orientation programs (Folsom, 1968). Some investigators question the appropriateness of reality orientation due to negative results reported from some studies (Zarit, 1986). Care was taken during orientation activities to prevent possible threat to esteem, considered by Schwartz (1974) to be the key to successful aging. Orientation occurred through visual stimuli of enlarged clocks, colorful signs, calendars and seasonal foods. Music was used with a subject's name and place of residence quoted in song verse. Attention was drawn to headlines in the newspaper, the weather, the date and day's events, and happenings of the past that occurred on the same date. Objects were provided for touching and feeling that encouraged orienting and increasing awareness to the environment. Exercises and sensory integration activity promoted body awareness. Cues to the present were provided throughout the program through conversation such as, "It seems hard to believe that tomorrow is 'Thanksgiving,'" or through props related to the season, e.g., a horn of plenty, pumpkin pie, or a story about the pilgrims. The concept behind this approach to reality orientation is that life must be interesting and fun with enough meaning and purpose to make it worthwhile to remain oriented. This belief is supported by Feil (1982) in her group work with the elderly.

The Multi-strategy program used some of the procedures found in Smith's remotivation program (Storandt, 1978). Ritual was established through specific happenings occurring routinely at the same time and place in the program. For example, socialization between residents and staff during refreshments occurred prior to establishing the climate of acceptance where each resident was welcomed with a warm hand shake and presented with his/her individualized name tag. As in the remotivation programs, preparation in the form of a pre planned topic with props was encouraged, but did not require adherence to the subject if the group led the discussion in another direction. In closing the session, appreciation was expressed for residents' attendance.

Sensory stimulation techniques (Richman, 1969, Burnside, 1970, 1974) were used in the Multi-strategy Program. Further support for their use was provided by Paire and Karney (1984). To assure sensory input, clear and slow speech, real flowers for touch and smell displayed on a white tablecloth, and familiar music with a pronounced rhythm were made a natural part of each program. Recognizing the diminished sensitivity of olfaction and gustation and the need to compensate for these losses during taste and smell stimulation, discussion and memories were used to reinforce the sensory experience (Myslinski, 1990).

Reminiscence as supported by many authorities (Butler and Lewis, 1973, Ebersole and Hess, 1981, and Edinberg, 1985) was incorporated into the Multi-strategy Program because of its flexibility, ease of application and tendency to occur naturally. Reminiscence was also used in the Multi-strategy Group as a tool for gaining knowledge and understanding about the older person and the period in which he/she had lived. It helped build a bridge between the past and present and create a path toward orientation.

Varied forms of exercise occurred in the Multi-strategy Program: breathing, stretching, broomstick, coordination, isometrics, and exercise through recreational activities or games requiring movement.

Music encouraged participation and helped increase or decrease the pace. Special attention was given in the Multi-strategy Program to pelvic floor exercises. Control of micturition and defecation may be enhanced through proprioceptive neuromuscular facilitation (Knott and Voss, 1968). Due to cognitive deficits of group members, an adaptation using sponges as props (under the feet and between the knees) helped achieve the desired muscle contractions. Kegel's or pelvic floor exercises are sometimes utilized for the same purpose (Wells, 1988). The theory that exercises are underutilized for preventing deterioration and improving respiratory and cardiovascular systems, body tone, strength, flexibility, and neuropsychologic and cognitive abilities was upheld by Powel (1974), Erickson (1978), Price and Luther (1980), Fiatarone and Evans (1990).

Touch, considered desirable by many authors (Montagu, 1978, Burnside, 1974, and Howard, 1988), was used through warm hand shakes, in assisting those needing help with exercises, during sensory stimulation activities and through holding hands with other residents during specific recreational games.

Rebuilding self esteem was carried out by drawing out, and recognizing talents, pointing out past achievements, and by encouraging listening to each other's stories, problems, and worries. Resident's names added to familiar songs or games such as "How-do-you do Mr. Jones" provided recognition and enjoyment. Members were offered choices in selections of activities and discussion topics. Topics such as religion, politics, and death, were not discouraged. (For example, in reverence for a member's death, a prayer or eulogy might be a part of the group program). Feelings and emotional memories were validated and each person was recognized as having wisdom from life experiences, thus assisting the regaining of dignity as suggested by Feil (1982, 1983). Talents, assets and strengths of subjects were discovered, increasing the group's respect for the individual.

Traditional Nursing Home Care

Traditional nursing home care is the kind of care usually found in nursing homes in this state. The settings where this study was conducted met with the minimum standards set by the federal and state government for care of residents in nursing homes. The programs offered by the facility were reality orientation, remotivation, exercises, educational activities, religious services, community outings, service projects, restorative nursing and physical therapy. Resident needs for involvement in these programs were determined through patient care planning sessions. No changes were made in determining the involvement or placement of the subjects within these groups, nor in their involvement in the activities normally taking place while providing them with their routine care. Eight hours of occupational therapy consultation took place monthly and the focus of work was guided by the nursing and activity directors. The emphasis was upon evaluations with recommendations for positioning, contracture prevention and feeding programs, using inservices related to care plans and meeting regulatory agency minimum standards.

RESULTS

Of the 72 subjects, 67 completed the study. Attrition left 34 subjects in the Multi-strategy Group and 33 in the Traditional Nursing Home Care Group. The average age of the subjects was 85.2 years for the Multi-strategy Group and 86.6 years for the Nursing Home Care Group. Table I shows the age characteristics for all the different categories in both groups. The Mann-Whitney U-Test was used to evaluate the difference in age between the Multi-strategy and the control group as well as the differences between these groups for the categories of mild, moderate, and severe organic brain syndrome. No significant difference was found.

The Wilcoxon Signed Rank Test was used to test Hypothesis I of no difference in pre and post scores on morale, mental function and activities of daily living for the Multi-strategy Group. When comparing the scores in each specific category of mild, moderate or severe organic brain syndrome, significant improvement between pre and post scores was found on morale, mental function and activities of daily living but not on the Face Hand Test. It should be noted in reading Table II that the Face-Hand Test and the Mental Status Questionnaire are error count scores and higher performance is indicated by a decrease in errors. As a whole, analysis showed a

CHARACTERISTICS OF MULTI-STRATEGY AND CONTROL GROUPS

	No. of Subjects in Multi-Strategy Group	Age Range of Multi-Strategy Group	Average Age of Multi Strategy Group	No. of Subjects in Control Group	Age Range of Control Group	Average Age of Control Group
Mild	11	72-92	84.2	9	72-98	86.
Moderate	12	80-89	85.6	12	81-96	87.8
Severe	11	81-92	85.8	12	73-98	84.7
Total	34	72-92	85.2	33	73-98	86.6

[a]Control Group refers to Traditional Nursing Home Care Groups

TABLE 1

141

COMPARISON OF PRE AND POST SCORES ON MORALE, MENTAL FUNCTION AND ACTIVITIES OF DAILY LIVING FOR MULTI-STRATEGY GROUP SUBJECTS[a]
(COMBINED CATEGORIES)

	Average Rank For Scores Which Decrease On Post Test	Average Rank For Scores Which Increase On Post Test	z[b]	P
Morale				
Total	0.0	16.0	-4.86	.001
Agitation	8.5	15.2	-4.52	.001
Attitude	6.5	13.3	-4.20	.001
Loneliness	8.2	16.8	-4.38	.001
Mental Functions				
Face-Hand Test	7.8	2.5	-2.83	.005
Mental Status Questionnaire	15.3	6.5	-4.56	.001
Activities of Daily Living	0.0	13.0	-4.37	.001

[a] n=34

[b] Wilcoxon Signed Rank Test

TABLE II

significant difference at better than the .005 level in pre and post test Multi-strategy Group measurements on morale, mental function and activities of daily living within the categories of mild, moderate and severe organic brain syndrome, and in all three groups combined. Table II illustrates the analysis for the combined categories. Hypothesis I was rejected.

Hypothesis II, stating no difference within the Traditional Nursing Home Care Group, used the same analysis. Overall, there was a significant difference on pre and post scores indicating lower scores in morale, mental function and activities of daily living for residents receiving traditional nursing home care only. Table III illustrates the analysis for the combined categories. Hypothesis II was rejected.

Hypothesis III, which states there would be no difference between the effects of the Multi-strategy Group Programs and the effects of traditional nursing home care within three categories of mild, moderate and severe organic brain syndrome and in the combined groups was also rejected. The Mann Whitney U-test was used to compare pre and post test scores of the two groups. There was no significant pre test difference between the two groups, nor between these two groups within the three categories of organic brain syndrome. The post test scores for the Multi-strategy Group were significantly better than for the Traditional Nursing Home Care Group, ($p < .03$) on all areas tested: morale, mental functioning and activities of daily living. Table IV illustrates the analysis for the combined categories.

DISCUSSION

The significant results of pre and post measurements $p < .005$ for the 34 subjects in the Multi-strategy Group may indicate that some residents diagnosed as having organic brain syndrome are "cast aside" without awareness of their potential for improvement. This is supported by Cohen and Eisdorfer (1985), who indicate that those who fit the labeling of organic brain syndrome, senile brain disease, dementia or Alzheimer's disease can improve in function with proper psychosocial treatment. This change was not limited to those with mild symptoms, but those with moderate and severe dysfunc-

COMPARISON OF PRE AND POST SCORES ON MORALE, MENTAL FUNCTION AND ACTIVITIES OF DAILY LIVING FOR SUBJECTS[a] RECEIVING TRADITIONAL NURSING HOME CARE (COMBINED CATEGORIES)

	Average Rank For Scores Which Decrease On Post Test	Average Rank For Scores Which Increase On Post Test	z[b]	p
Morale				
Total	14.5	8.3	-4.14	.001
Agitation	7.9	7.0	-0.65	NS
Attitude	11.6	7.5	-3.23	.001
Loneliness	12.2	7.3	-3.39	.001
Mental Function				
Face-Hand Test	6.4	8.8	-1.59	NS
Mental Status Questionnaire	0.0	6.5	-3.06	.002
Activities of Daily Living	10.9	9.2	-2.20	.028

[a] n=33

[b] Wilcoxon Signed Rank Test

TABLE III

COMPARISON OF SUBJECTS IN MULTI-STRATEGY GROUP VS. TRADITIONAL
CARE GROUP ON PRE AND POST MORALE, MENTAL FUNCTION, AND
ACTIVITIES OF DAILY LIVING
(COMBINED CATEGORIES)

	Multi-Strategy Group Mean Rank (n=34)	Traditional Care Group Mean Rank (n=33)	Mann Whitney U[a]	P
Morale				
Total				
Pre	31.7	36.4	483.5	NS
Post,	45.7	21.9	164.5	.001
Agitation				
Pre	31.4	36.7	472.5	NS
Post	39.7	28.2	369.0	.013
Attitude				
Pre	32.6	35.5	512.0	NS
Post	45.2	22.4	179.0	.001
Loneliness				
Pre	31.7	36.4	482.0	NS
Post	45.4	22.2	173.0	.001
Mental Function				
Face-Hand Test				
Pre	33.2	34.8	534.5	NS
Post	28.8	39.4	384.5	.025
Mental Status Questionnaire				
Pre	32.6	35.5	513.0	NS
Post	25.1	43.2	258.0	.001
Activities of Daily Living				
Pre	33.8	34.2	555.0	NS
Post	39.1	28.8	388.5	.03

[a]Corrected for ties   TABLE IV

tion also improved significantly. Many factors discussed below
may relate to or account for the improvement in residents who received the Multi-strategy Program.

Recognizing the detrimental effects to residents of having staff
with misconceptions related to aging, four one hour inservices were

provided the leaders prior to starting the Multi-strategy Program. Their brief introduction to psychosocial theories and concepts such as the spiral of senility and myths of aging helped the leaders have a more positive attitude toward their work and improved their relationship with residents.

The occupational therapist also provided a weekly inservice to the leaders to direct the individualization of each resident's needs and assets to the specific program strategies. The focus was upon the whole person concept of treatment (Kirchman, 1986), using techniques for minimizing and compensating for losses, creating an environment of respect, and supporting or improving the group members competence and esteem.

Consistent attendance at the regularly scheduled Multi-strategy Programs provided added structure to the residents' lives. Combined with the pleasure connected with the program there was a reason for being oriented and a purpose for performing activities of daily living in preparation for attendance at the group meetings.

It is believed that improved self esteem brought the desire to reflect the renewed self image and this impacted upon the improvement in activities of daily living scores. The leaders were instructed on precautionary measures and exercise techniques to enhance performance in residents with arthritis, strokes, and Parkinson's disease. It is believed that the dulling of individual sensory reception due to immobilization and confinement in a nursing home was reversed as emphasis was placed upon voluntary movement even within the confines of a wheelchair. The proprioceptive input provided by exercise and activities within the program prevented further physical deterioration and intellectual dulling.

The structure of this program allowed the leader to use his/her personality and creativity. The leader, having basic knowledge of reality orientation, remotivation, reminiscence, was encouraged to use activities and approaches in which he/she felt most comfortable. The structure was loose enough to be adaptable to the many levels of residents' function, and encouraged their use as "helpers" in leading some portions of the program. There was enough variety of activity to allow the worker to choose what felt most suitable. Artificiality did not develop. This may happen easily in programs such as reality orientation and remotivation (Storandt, 1978). The freedom to include variety within the program seemed to prevent boredom of the leader and tended to foster increased interest and orientation of the group.

The following observations not only support the interpretation of the statistical finding, but also indicate that staff were encouraged to have greater interest in their work. After a few weeks of attendance in the group, one resident who had little concern about her appearance and was always observed sitting slumped over in a chair, requested help in fixing her hair, attempted to fix her own dress, and asked if someone could help her find a new one to wear to the meetings. Nursing aides observing the Multi-strategy Program were overheard saying that they did not know that Mr. Jones ever smiled before, and another commented that they all seemed to be having such a good time. It was gratifying to one of the activity workers to have one of the men thank her each day for inviting him to the meetings.

In contrast, the traditional nursing home programs showed some inherent weaknesses. The fact that the study showed the 33 subjects in the Traditional Care Group to have significant decrease in morale, mental function, and activities of daily living should raise questions related to the spiral of senility, social breakdown syndrome, sensory deprivation and decreasing esteem. Some of the programs, such as Reality Orientation, in the traditional group, were carried out by the same staff that carried out the Multi-strategy Groups, therefore it is unlikely that the charisma of leaders effected the results. The focus of the problem related to inconsistent scheduling of programs, infrequent evaluations and recommendations by an occupational therapist, and staff's poor follow up to achieve goals. As supported by Storandt (1978), the procedures for carrying out programs (such as reality orientation and remotivation) are often drastically changed and are not implemented in the manner intended by the originators. Reality orientation was not scheduled daily nor was the necessary training provided to carry out 24 hour reality orientation. In observing the approach to classroom orientation of residents, the request for rote repetition of materials increased residents' awareness of their cognitive loss, thus decreasing esteem and increasing withdrawal. Also, the author observed that patient care planning sessions were carried out hurriedly with the intent of fulfilling the need for completed paper work required by the federal and state regulations, and the actual involvement of a resident in programs was not carried out as set down in the plans. More attention was given to the offering of programs to meet requirements than to the examination of resident's reason for active or non participation in programs. Although many programs were offered, many were passive entertainment. They did not offer the opportunity for a cohesive group in which residents could develop a sense of belonging.

Lack of stimulation may also have been a factor in bringing about the significant decrease between pre and post scores of the control group. It is the author's belief that subjects in the control group spent too much idle time in retrospection, in sitting, often confined, or lying down. Strength and agility can be lost in far less time than four months, and if the residents perceived helplessness it can cause irreversible damage (Henry, 1986). The optimal level of stimulation required for arousal, positive affective tone, cognitive and motor activity may not have been occurring in this group. Without the daily intense effort by staff to explore assets, give recognition for past talents, provide the opportunity to contribute to a group and develop a sense of belonging and self esteem, the traditional nursing home care residents were at risk for being categorized as helpless and hopeless and perceiving themselves as deficient and incompetent. None of the traditional nursing home care group programs were provided daily, therefore the structure that was provided by the Multi-strategy Group was missing.

The "Spiral of Senility" described by Barns (1976) was in progress, and without appropriate intervention the subjects in the Traditional Care Group were becoming closer to vegetation and death. Activities that improve self esteem were not consistently utilized, and depressive symptoms or organic brain syndrome symptoms that can be addressed with nonpharmacological approaches according to Frengley (1987), were not of sufficient magnitude to provide improvement in function. As decline in functioning was realized, there was a decrease in morale and self-esteem.

By contrasting methods used with both groups, the strengths of the Multi-strategy Group and the weaknesses in the Traditional

Nursing Home Care Group, a rationale for the results of the research is presented.

CONCLUSION

The study supports the use of a Multi-strategy Program for residents with symptoms of organic brain syndrome. It showed an increase in morale, mental function and activities of daily living following four months of Multi-strategy Program intervention and a decrease in these areas for the control group. Further study of the value of various programs used in nursing homes is needed and an effort to identify those most cost effective would be appropriate. It is recommended that a replication of this study occur, and that more work be done to determine the psychosocial aspects of senile dementia, and the effects of sensory deprivation in the elderly.

REFERENCES

Bach, J., Zarit, S., Miller, C. A., & Tang, J. K. (1988). An autopsy research program. *American Journal of Alzheimer's Care*. 3 (2) 9-14.

Barns, E., Sack, A., Shore, H. (1973). Guidelines to treatment approaches. *Gerontologist*, 8, 513-527.

Bender, M. B. (1952). *Disorders in Perception*. Springfield, Illinois: Charles C Thomas.

Bender, M. B. (1975). Incidence and types of perceptual deficiencies in the aged. In W. S. Fields (Ed.) *Neurological and Sensory Disorders in the Elderly*. New York: Stratton International Medical Books Corporation.

Bondareff, W. (1986). Biomedical perspective of Alzheimer's disease and dementia in the elderly. In, Mary L. M. Gilhooly, S. H. Zarit & J. E. Birren, (Eds.), *The Dementias: Policy and Management*. Englewood Cliffs, NJ: Prentice-Hall.

Burnside, I. M. (1970). Clocks and calendars, *American Journal of Nursing*, 70 (1).

Burnside, I. M. (1974). Sensory stimulation with regressed aged patients. *American Journal of Nursing*.

Bussee, E. W., & Pfeiffer, E. (1977). *Behavior and Adaptation in Late Life*. Boston: Little, Brown & Co.

Butler, R. N., & Lewis, M. I. (1973). *Aging and Mental Health*. Saint Louis: C.V. Mosby Company.

Cohen, D., & E., Carl. (1986). *The Loss of Self*, New York: W. W. Norton & Company.

Congressional Summary. (1987). *Losing a million minds*. U. S. Government Printing Office, Washington DC.

Ebersole, P., & Hess, P. (1981). *Toward healthy aging*, St. Louis: C. V. Mosby, Co.

Edinberg, M. A. (1985). *Mental health practice with the elderly*, New Jersey: Prentice-Hall.

Eisdorfer, C., and Cohen, D., (1978). The cognitively impaired elderly: Differential diagnosis, In M. Storandt & I. Siegler, & M. Elias (Eds.). *The clinical psychology of aging*. New York, Plenum Press.

Ernst, P., Beran, B., Safford, F., & Kleinhauz, M. (1978). Isolation and the symptoms of organic brain syndrome. *Gerontologist* 18 (5) 468-474.

Fabiszewiski, K. J., Riley, M. E., Berkley, D, Karner, J. & Shea, S. (1988). Management of advanced Alzheimer's dementia, In L. Volicer, K. Fabiszewski, Y. Rheaume, K. Lasch. (Eds.). *Clinical management of Alzheimer's Disease*. Rockville, Maryland: Aspen Publishers.

Feil, Naomi (1983). Groupwork with disoriented nursing home residents. In S. Shura (Ed.). *Groupwork with the frail elderly*. New York: The Haworth Press, Inc.

Fiatarone, M. A., Evans, W. (1990). Exercises in the oldest old. *Geriatric Rehabilitation*, 5 (2) 66-77.

Folsom, J. C. (1968). Reality orientation for the elderly mental ill. *Journal of Geriatric Psychiatry* 1 (2).

Frengley, Dermot J. (1989). Depression, In Generations, *Journal of American Society Aging*, (XII) 1. 29-33.

Goldfarb, A. I., (1974). *Aging and organic brain syndrome: Recognizing the problem*, Fort Washington, PA: McNeil Laboratories, Inc.

Gotestam, K. Kunnar, (1980). Behavior and dynamic psychotherapy with the elderly, In J. E., Birren & R. B. Sloane (Eds.). *Handbook of mental health and aging*. Englewood Cliffs, NJ: Prentice-Hall, Inc. pp 775-804.

Helmick, C. E., Henry, M. E., Aubert, R. E., Gurber, T. M., & Sayetta, R. B. (1988). State surveillance of dementing illnesses; perspective and workshop recommendations. *American Journal of Alzheimer's Care*. 3 (5) 40-45.

Henry, James, P. (1986). Relation of psychosocial factors to the senile dementias. In M. L. Gilhooly, S. Zarit, & J. E. Birren, (Eds.). *The Dementias; policy & management*, New Jersey: Prentice-Hall.

Howard, Deborah M. (1988). The effects of touch in the geriatrics. *Physical & Occupational Therapy Journal of Research*. (6), 2, 35-47.

Kahn, R. L. (1971). Psychological aspects of aging. In Rossman, I. (Ed.). *Clinical geriatrics*. Philadelphia: J. B. Lippincott.

Kahn, R. N. & Miller, N. E. (1978). Assessment of altered brain function in the aged. In M. Storandt, I. Seigler & M. I. Elias (Eds.) *Clinical psychology of aging*. New York, Plenum Press.

Kern, Donald C., (1988). Epidemiology and Prevention of Alzheimer's Disease. In L. Volicer, K.J. Fabiszewski, Y. L. Rheaume, K. E. Lasch (Eds.). *Clinical management of Alzheimer's disease*, Rockville, Maryland, Aspen Publisher.

Kirchman, M. M. (1986). Measuring the quality of life. *Occupational Therapy Journal of Research*. 6 (1), 21-32.

Knott, M. & Voss, D. (1968). *Proprioceptive neuromuscular facilitation: patterns and techniques*. New York, Harper and Row, Hoeber Medical Division.

Lawton, P.M. (1975). The Philadelphia geriatric center morale scale: A revision. *Journal of Gerontology*, 30 (1). 85-89.

Levy, L. (1986). A practical guide to the care of Alzheimer's disease victims: The cognitive disability perspective, *Topics in Geriatric Rehabilitation*, 1, 16-22.

Montagu, A., (1978). *Touching: the human significance of the skin*, New York: Harper & Row.

Oster, C. (1976). Sensory deprivation in geriatric patients. *Journal American Geriatric Society*, 10.

Parent, L. H. (1978). Effects of low stimulus environment on behavior. *American Journal of Occupational Therapy*, 32 (1).

Paire, J. A. & Karney, R. J. (1984). The effectiveness of sensory stimulation for geropsychiatric inpatients. *American Journal of Occupational Therapy*, 38. 505-509.

Powell, R. R. (1974). Psychological effects of exercise therapy upon institutional geriatric patients. *Journal of Gerontology* 29: 157-161.

Reichenbach, Velma Russ. (1981). Thesis, Occupational Therapy Department, University of Illinois, Chicago.

Richman, L. (1969). Sensory training in treatment of geriatric patients. *American Journal of Occupational Therapy*. 23: 254-257.

Storandt, Martha. (1978). Other approaches to therapy, In M. Storandt, I. Siegler, & E. Merrill, *The clinical psychology of aging*, (pp 277-293), New York, Plenum Press.

Swartz, A. N. (1974). An observation on self-esteem as the linchpin of quality of life for the aged. *A training manual covering the psychosocial dimensions of care in long term care facilities*. Los Angeles, Ethel Percy Andrus Gerontology Center, 1974.

Wells, Thelma I., Additional treatment for urinary incontinence, *Topics in Geriatric Rehabilitation*, 3 (2) 48-57.

Zarit, Steven H. & Anthony, Cheri R. (1986). Interventions with dementia patients and their families, In M. Gilhooly, S. Zarit, & J. E. Birren (Eds.) *The dementias: policy and management*. New Jersey: Prentice-Hall.

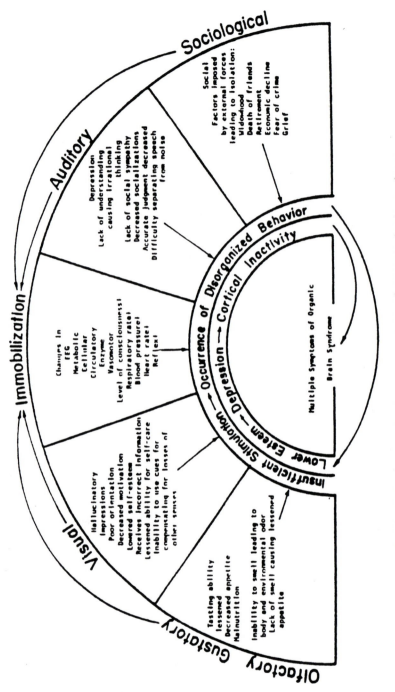

Deprivation factors leading to symptoms of organic brain syndrome.

APPENDIX A

Reichenbach, (1981)

Program Planning
in Geriatric Psychiatry:
A Model
for Psychosocial Rehabilitation

Danielle N. Butin, OTR, MPH
Colleen Heaney, BS, MA

SUMMARY. The psychosocial rehabilitation model described in this article demonstrates the effectiveness of therapeutic activity disciplines collaborating and working together. Several assessment tools, common skill acquisition needs and models of individual and group interventions are discussed.

Psychosocial rehabilitation in geriatric psychiatry is based on the premise that success in self-care, leisure and work is crucial to mental well being. The objective of program planning is to comprehensively assess function and to promote optimal performance in areas of cognition, interpersonal skills, self-care, leisure, work, and utilization of community resources. Maintaining levels of activity involvement with adaptability and flexibility is an essential component of late life satisfaction. The geriatric activity program at the New York Hospital is a comprehensive rehabilitation model that positively impacts on patients' well-being.

Danielle N. Butin is Occupational Therapist in the Geriatric Services Division at The New York Hospital, Cornell Medical Center-Westchester Division, White Plains, NY and Coordinator of the Maturity Curriculum for the Department of Occupational Therapy at Dominican College, Blauvelt, NY.

Colleen Heaney is Program Coordinator of Therapeutic Activities in the Geriatric Services Division at The New York Hospital, Cornell Medical Center-Westchester Division, White Plains, NY.

Please address correspondence to both authors at: 21 Bloomingdale Road, White Plains, NY 10605.

The Westchester Division of the New York Hospital-Cornell Medical Center is a university based non-profit voluntary psychiatric facility. The 322 bed inpatient clinical service has a separate division of geriatric services, with three units totaling 66 beds.

Separate departments of medicine, nursing, social work, psychology, and therapeutic activities comprise the multi-disciplinary team. Three of the five therapeutic activity professionals who treat geriatric patients are represented on each unit, and serve as case managers for their patients. The arbitrary age for admission to the geriatric service is 55 with potential range from 55-98 years old. The average length of stay is five weeks. Though a wide variety of neurological and psychiatric disorders are represented, the majority of patients are admitted for diagnosis and treatment of an affective disorder or an organic mood disturbance. Diagnosis, prognosis, chronological age and expected discharge environment often do not influence placement on any particular unit because bed availability is an over-riding concern. Those persons with affective disorders, dementia, or long term chronic psychiatric illness may live on the same unit.

The wide variation in developmental and chronological age for this heterogenous group, and the brief length of stay presented a significant challenge to activity program planning and treatment. Equally challenging for activity rehabilitation is that a medical model of treatment prevails, and in the past, psycho-social rehabilitation had been minimized or disregarded. Elderly patients, family members and many professional staff readily abdicated all clinical decisions to professionals, and symptom relief was seen as the ultimate answer. Prior to aggressive efforts to restructure activity rehabilitation, geriatric patients were treated biologically, received individual and family therapy, and participated in a largely diversional activity program. The patients generally were discharged free of major psychiatric symptomatology and were given a suggested aftercare plan. However, maladaptive behavior patterns and skill dysfunction that can accompany mental illness or result from loss of esteem and confidence was manifest throughout the hospitalization and evident at discharge. Patients were often at risk for non-compliance in following discharge recommendations, were unsuccessful in adapting to their discharge environment, and were risks for recidivism.

Over the past five years, the authors have worked extensively to develop a program that would more definitively address psychosocial aspects of rehabilitation and challenge patients, families and staff to acknowledge the importance of it. The complexion of professonal staff in the Geriatrics Therapeutic Activity Division include a gerontological counselor, an occupational therapist, two recreational therapists, and a creative arts therapist. A liaison vocational counselor is also available for those persons who have work as a priority goal. Through collaborative efforts of these professionals, a framework for treatment has been established that uses counseling techniques to promote purposeful involvement in activity. Activity rehabilitation has gradually, but consistently become integrated into treatment in the geriatric division, and is currently recognized as tantamount to recovering from mental illness.

FRAME OF REFERENCE

Although the disengagement theory suggests that older people naturally become more self-involved and less interested in others or external events, clinical observations and scientific studies dispute this view of universal disengagement (Neugarten, 1965, Havighurst, 1968). Disengagement theorists claim that this reaction is a response to inner needs and not a response to socio-cultural pressure (Cummings, 1961). A universal disengagement process is an overgeneralization, and lacks the consideration and integration of an individual's lifestyle as a predictor of successful aging (Neugarten, 1965). In fact, social involvements and commitments are the factors most strongly associated with well-being during the natural adjustment to old age. Greater life satisfaction has been found amongst seniors who are active in both community activities and family roles. Since life satisfaction is more closely related to levels of activity than inactivity, older adults who maintain greater amounts of activity report high levels of gratification and contentment (Havighurst, 1961). Activity theory stresses the need for older adults to maintain active involvement and to augment and replace activities to assure continued satisfaction and mental well-being (Pikunas, 1969). Older adults age favorably if they remain active, cope with major life losses, and find meaningful replacement activities for those relinquished. Generally, older adults have the same psycho-social needs as middle aged adults, with the exception of biological and health related changes (Havighurst, 1961).

As older people age, however, activity levels may decrease with restrictive opportunities for interpersonal pursuits. Life satisfaction tends to be greater when physical and mental health states are sound (Maddox, 1965). People limited in activities of daily living, access to community services and vocational opportunities are least likely to report feeling satisfied and fulfilled (Smith, 1972). Psychogeriatric patients are frequently faced with the dual burden of coping with a major psychiatric disorder, while attempting to adapt to physical changes and limitations. Skills in carrying out activities of daily living, working or volunteering at a relatively satisfying job, enjoying avocational and creative pursuits, and relating interpersonally are frequently impaired amongst psychiatric patients (Mosey, 1970).

The overall goal of psychiatric rehabilitation is to promote patient satisfaction and provide learning opportunities for the skills necessary to accomplish tasks of everyday living (Fidler, 1984). The necessary components for a meaningful activity program for older adults with psychiatric illness are sensory stimulation and reality orientation for the cognitively impaired or severely regressed; remotivation for patients who are socially withdrawn and alienated from their surroundings but capable of coherent interactions and able to perform graded simple tasks; complex and challenging activities for those whose social and functional skills are relatively intact; transitional activities or volunteer work to meet the needs of those returning home with community responsibilities (Weiner, 1978).

Following initial assessments of their needs, capabilities, and wishes for rehabilitation, patients are referred for individual or group treatment. This process encourages skill development and incremental progress toward attainment of individualized activity goals that are vital to the well being of the elderly patient.

ASSESSMENTS

Comprehensive assessments are the cornerstone of psychosocial treatment in the geriatric division. These assessments help determine assets and liabilities in cognition, interpersonal skills, task performance, physical ability, leisure and social involvement and utilization of community resources. The assessments guide treatment, maximize individualized interventions and promote programming that is responsive to the expressed interests of each patient.

The rehabilitation process is initiated (within a few days of admission), when the Therapeutic Activities Representative meets with the patient and engages him/her in a planning dialogue. The Rehabilitation Activity Assessment helps determine the patient's overall goals in self-care, work, and leisure and elicits participation in identifying and prioritizing skills and behaviors needed to attain their goals. Patients who have the cognitive skills to participate meaningfully in this process value this tool as it promotes participation in a rehabilitation plan that is self-generated. This model gives patients the opportunity to identify goals, determine needed skills, select methods for skill acquisition and augment or modify their goals in relationship to their ongoing performance.

Sometimes the patients are seriously cognitively impaired, or too psychiatrically ill to realistically determine their goals and needs. In these cases, the Therapeutic Activity Representative provides assistance in referring to groups and recommending discharge plans that are consistent with their needs for support.

Consistent application of this initial dialogue with geriatric patients has generated some common rehabilitation goals and skills needed to achieve the goals. Individual and group treatment that reflects the patient's priority needs in self-care, work or leisure and focuses on their level of functioning have been conceptualized with regard to the patient's expressed interest for rehabilitation.

Self-care treatment generally focuses on skills needed for the patient to manage in their living environment following discharge. Treatment in the leisure category addresses the skills needed for the patient to spend free time qualitatively. Treatment in the work category focuses on skills needed to resume paid employment or acquire a volunteer job. Some common examples of overall rehabilitation goals and required skills in these areas are as follows.

Self-Care Rehabilitation Goals

1. I will go to a nursing home when I am discharged from the hospital.
2. I want to move to my daughter's house when I leave the hospital.
3. I want to return home to my apartment when I am discharged from the hospital.

SKILLS:
- identifying self-care strengths and weaknesses
- improving attention to hygiene
- following schedule
- improving nutritional awareness
- managing money
- accepting help from a home health aide
- managing transportation
- cooking and meal planning
- expressing opinions
- tolerating others
- improving confidence
- expressing satisfaction
- following routine
- researching residences

Leisure Rehabilitation Goals

1. I want to participate in the activity program at the nursing home when I am discharged.
2. I want to find people to play bridge with in my location when I leave the hospital.
3. I want to join a senior center when I leave the hospital.

SKILLS:
- clarifying current and past leisure interests
- enriching or renewing leisure interests
- improving skill in a leisure activity
- finding community leisure options

- increasing confidence and independence in using community resources
- initiating leisure involvements
- initiating contacts with peers

Work Rehabilitation Goals

1. I want to be productive in my nursing home environment.
2. I want to find a volunteer job in the community when I leave the hospital.
3. I want to find paid employment in the community when I leave the hospital.

SKILLS:
- clarifying work/volunteer history and aspirations
- identifying concerns regarding retirement
- improving awareness of post-retirement options
- accepting supervision in the work setting
- increasing willingness to accept challenge and responsibility in work setting
- working cooperatively with others
- organizing tasks
- increasing productivity in tasks
- exploring community services
- interviewing for job
- identifying work related skills

The described assessment and planning dialogue almost always signals a need for additional assessments to supplement, validate or help patients measure the congruence between their goals, assests and liabilities.

The SHORT-CARE (Comprehensive Assessment and Referral Evaluation) (Gurland, 1984) is often used to gather additional functional information. The SHORT-CARE discourages reliance on typical symptoms only for resolution of psychiatric illness. It encourages a probing look at the etiology of specific areas of psychosocial dysfunction. This standardized, multidimensional semi-structured interview provides clinicians with scales for depression, dementia, and disability. The SHORT-CARE assists therapists in becoming more cognizant of each patient's individual needs for rehabilitation and aftercare.

Patients are also assessed with the Activities Health Assessment. This tool provides both therapists and patients with information about time management, involvement in meaningful activities, and discharge planning.

Finally, patients are constantly assessed and observed while participating in functional activities. They have opportunities to critique their own performance while receiving feedback about the specific skills needed to attain their overall rehabilitation goal.

PROGRAM DESCRIPTION

The primary objective of activity rehabilitation in geriatrics is to help each patient identify their specific goals and needed skills in self-care, leisure and work. Because the therapeutic activity professionals recognize the broad range of dysfunction, there is commitment to meeting individual needs. The program and the therapists are highly flexible while maintaining a core structure that provides stability. This is accomplished by offering groups that closely parallel the expected plans for the individual's discharge environment. It is also accomplished by expecting the therapist to individualize treatment within the context of the group. For example, in a verbal group, one patient may be working on expressing opinions, while another patient might be working on the acquisition of listening skills because they are dominant interrupters. A moderately demented patient might cook in a group with patients preparing for discharge because they have maintained a skill in that one area.

Groups are generally organized with regard for the patient's functional status and need for different amounts of support. This assures successful involvements while challenging the patient to continually use skills that have been neglected.

After assessments are completed, findings are collected and analyzed. The patients are then referred to groups that can provide them with skill acquisition that they, or the therapist, has determined as essential for success in their discharge environment. Patients are given large print schedules with a detailed description of groups. The schedules have a space for the therapist and patient to list the specific skills requiring attention within the context of each group. Since each group has a clearly defined protocol, therapists are aware of the specific guidelines and objectives for that group. As an example, the Leisure Planning Protocol is described in Table 1.

Each program cluster (self-care, work and leisure) has groups that respond to the requirement for maximum, moderate or minimum levels of support. As patients improve or plateau they are encouraged to participate in increasingly challenging activities. Examples of the program are provided to illustrate how assessment findings are applied to the level of support needed in group treatment.

GROUP STRUCTURE OFFERING MAXIMUM SUPPORT

Patient Population

This population is quite regressed due to depression, chronic schizophrenia, or dementia, and is moderately to severely cognitively impaired. They are alert, but frequently disoriented. If their level of function remains the same throughout hospitalization, these patients are usually discharged to an institutional facility, or return home with significant home care, and a structured day program.

Self-Care

Assistance and encouragement is needed in all activities of daily living, and patients are unable to follow simple 1-2 step directions. Decisions do not show good judgement and supervision is required to maintain safety. These are patients who have a limited investment in how they look, how they spend their time, and often deny, minimize or overlook difficulties.

SELF-CARE SKILLS:
- Following simple directions while grooming
- Eating independently
- Dressing with minimal cuing and encouragement
- Finding room on the unit
- Using notes to compensate for memory problems

TABLE 1. Leisure Planning Protocol

<u>Days</u>: M-W-F   <u>Time</u>: 1:30 - 2:45PM

PROBLEMS	SHORT TERM GOALS
1. Patient unable to identify leisure interests.	1. Patient will identify one or two interests within the group.
2. Patient unable to independently plan or participate in meaningful activities.	2. Patient will cooperatively plan and participate in one community activity per week with peers on the unit.
3. Patient is unaware of leisure resources or how to access these services in the community.	3. Patient will call two or three community resources per week to heighten awareness or available programs.

LONG TERM GOALS

1. Patient will commit to two-three community based activities based on identified interests.

----

2. Patient will initiate suggestions and plans for weekly community outing.

----

3. Patient will develop a resource file of meaningful activities in the community prior to discharge.

INTERVENTIONS

1. Identifying Leisure Interests Leader provides leisure interest finders and value surveys to encourage identification and exploration of interests.

----

2. Planning Leader encourages group to cooperatively identify and plan one community activity. Patients utilize resource file to make arrangements and calls.

----

3. Implementation Leader accompanies group on the community trip. patients secure names on mailing lists and independently seek out information for their involvement.

Leisure

Activity participation is limited. They cannot generate interests or skills, and require constant encouragement and stimulation to remain engaged in purposeful activity. They minimally communicate with each other, and are withdrawn and isolative.

LEISURE SKILLS: • Attempting an adapted version of an activity from the past
• Tolerating the presence of others
• Initiating and completing a task within one group setting

Work

Patients are unable to work productively in organizing tasks to completion. They are easily frustrated and have no tolerance for stress. Difficulties sequencing logical steps in an organized manner are noted.

WORK SKILLS: • Asking for clarification or assistance
• Maintaining participation in task activities for 15 minute periods
• Sequencing simple steps in a logical order
• Following simple directions

Activity groups organized for this population illustrate ways to engage the seriously regressed geriatric population. The severely regressed begin each day with sensory stimulation and exercise. Old familiar show tunes lead even the most regressed patient through pleasurable movements. Balloon volleyball ends this daily session with increased alertness and heightened sensitivity to the environment.

Simple repetitive tasks are provided to encourage basic responsibility for one's immediate environment. Examples of volunteer jobs on the unit include folding laundry, ringing meal bell, dusting tables, and changing tablecloths. Jobs are listed weekly on the unit bulletin board, with the patient's name, and cuing is provided consistently by the inter-disciplinary team.

Many strategies of an adaptive function model are incorporated in the remotivation group. Modalities utilized to increase socialization, and sensitivity to the immediate environment are memory games, elder trivia, reminiscent slide shows, pet therapy, nature outings, murals, improvisation, and simple baking.

For the more regressed, individual work includes sensory stimulation, and in some cases holding stuffed animals has been therapeutic.

GROUP STRUCTURE OFFERING MODERATE SUPPORT

Patient Population

This population represents those older adults with partial symptom resolution following biological, milieu, activity and counseling therapies. As patients improve, they need new challenges. Although they are alert and oriented, they may be mildly cognitively impaired, and still depressed. If their condition remains stable, they are usually discharged to a senior residence, or home with senior day treatment. Moderate support is required because the therapist must organize components of their projects, while encouraging greater self-reliance amongst group members. The leader encourages interaction, and promotes opportunities for group feedback, but must continue to be the facilitator.

Self-Care

Although needing help with problem solving, most can perform activities of daily living with minimal assistance. They are able to recognize areas of difficulty and may begin to ask for help and feedback.

SELF-CARE SKILLS:
- Following activity schedule independently
- Participating in meal planning and preparation
- Making bed
- Cleaning bedroom
- Organizing datebook with telephone numbers and appointments

Leisure

Interest and motivation for leisure involvements is inconsistent. They initiate activities within structured settings, but not outside of group opportunities. These are people who have difficulty asking peers to join them for a casual activity or conversation. They are dependent on a group leader for initiating interaction, and rarely generate involvement independently.

LEISURE SKILLS: • Setting up supplies needed for a group activity
 • Attending all scheduled activities
 • Identifying interests to pursue upon discharge

Work

Patients derive genuine pleasure from involvement in work-related projects, or commitments that improve the lives of others. They continue to rely on group leader for directions and instructions to follow-through on tasks appropriately.

WORK SKILLS: • Identifying ways to remain committed to meaningful work-related activity
 • Improving investment in quality of work
 • Increasing confidence in familiar tasks

Patients in this phase of treatment are expected to be familiar with unit and activity routines. They often begin their day with discussion of current events, and are encouraged to bring at least one or more topics of interest to the group. This intervention provides them with a non-threatening way to participate in discussions.

Often patients demonstrate increased independence by participating in a cooking group. By making snacks for their unit, and initiating luncheons for peers, family members, staff or guests, they begin to regain confidence in a wide range of skills. A leisure skills group provides an opportunity to get acquainted with peers who share similar interests. Group leaders facilitate opportunities for patients who value bridge, Scrabble™, shuffleboard, to know one another and make commitments. This is important for those who will return to a center, because they will be expected to initiate and join social activities.

Finally, exposure to volunteer activity is popular at this phase of treatment. Community service projects help patients move outside themselves and offer something to others. This group has frequently made and contributed toys to homeless children, participated in clerical tasks needed for fund raising events, maintained bulletin boards, designed advertisement flyers and contributed information to the patients' newsletter. The leader usually needs to provide tasks, direction and encouragement.

GROUP STRUCTURE OFFERING MINIMUM SUPPORT

Patient Population

This group is approaching discharge and has resolved a major depressive disorder. After a major depression has been treated with medication, maladaptive behaviors are often apparent. Patients continue to struggle with dependency; helplessness; anger over losses; and poor coping mechanisms. They can use insight oriented experiences to understand maladaptive patterns and initiate and practice alternate coping mechanisms. This population generally returns home with a clearly defined plan to pursue for community involvement. The therapist encourages increased leadership and opportunities for problem solving by operationalizing decisions made within the group, and helping members to see the carryover process. Although they are cognitively intact and usually physically healthy, they frequently have lifelong difficulties with adaptation, making and keeping friends, and interacting meaningfully in the community. They need careful individualized programs to help compensate for life-long problems reaching out for help.

Self-Care

Any limitations in activities of daily living are minimized because of fears of dependency. They struggle with issues of interdependence, and lack the ability to comfortably ask for help. Familiar tasks, like cooking or balancing a checkbook, are resisted because of anxiety or lack of familiarity with the task (following the death of a spouse). Some self-care tasks may be difficult due to dependency and anxiety.

SELF-CARE SKILLS:
- Planning and ordering food for meals
- Arranging transportation for passes
- Practicing asking for help
- Identifying strengths in self-care

Leisure

Although motivated and interested in meaningful activities, they need encouragement and support to participate in new or challenging activities. They are quite anxious about engaging in community outings and returning home.

LEISURE SKILLS:
- Identifying activities to pursue upon discharge
- Participating in a few community outings per week
- Planning and arranging details for community based activities
- Asking peers to participate in unstructured activities
- Initiating meaningful activities during unstructured time

Work

They are motivated to translate interests into community service or employment. These skills are practiced while hospitalized and only assistance with major decisions is needed.

WORK SKILLS:
- Identifying specific volunteer/paid employment interests
- Practicing skills needed for expected job
- Exploring community options for work
- Arranging details and interviews
- Identifying strengths and deficits

This population is approaching discharge to the community following treatment for a major depression. Generally, they have reacquired essential concrete skills, but maladaptive behaviors may resurface or continue to be apparent as the patient faces discharge without the intense support they had during hospitalizaton. Struggles with dependency, anger over losses, fears of incompetence and interpersonal problems are highlighted as expectations for more challenging functioning is indicated. Essential in this phase of treatment are opportunities to verbally express concerns and get support, but shift emphasis away from the activity therapist and toward themselves and others. Counseling groups that focus on increased autonomy, choice, and responsibility are introduced along with more challenging activities. These interventions help patients to identify concerns, explore coping strategies and practice activities designed to rekindle feelings of competence and worthwhileness.

The Leisure Planning Group is a three part group that helps older adults identify interests, community events, and plan a weekly community outing. An extensive file of community resources is available. Group participants are expected to make appropriate calls and arrangements.

Goals Group uses activity and cognitive therapy models to empower and assist in re-gaining some control and mastery of life tasks. The action oriented verbal-task group stresses exploration of coping and problem solving skills, emphasizes collaborative involvement and encourages goal directed activity that alters the person's role from that of subordinate to peer group member responsible to themselfs and others. Homework is given and participants are encouraged to practice specific strategies to optimize their independence in preparation for discharge.

To practice better communicating strategies with their grandchildren, an intergenerational meal group was established in collaboration with hospitalized adolescents. An older adult patient was matched with an adolescent to foster and learn appropriate interactive strategies to carryover at home. The dyads inter-changed responsibilities for meal planning, and each dyad assumed responsibility for the preparation of specific components of the meal. Older patients used past meal planning skills, while practicing appropriate interactive styles necessary for healthy relationships at home.

For those patients who have work as a priority goal, Vocational Services provides them with opportunities for volunteer jobs throughout the hospital. The placement is viewed as a vital reality testing tool. Examples of volunteer jobs used by hospitalized older adults have included a plant operations director volunteering in the hospital maintenance department, a retired secretary volunteering as a research librarian, and a knitting teacher volunteering as an instructor with older and younger long term patients.

CONCLUSION

The geriatric psycho-social rehabilitation program has become well regarded and integrated into the fabric of comprehensive, multi-disciplinary treatment.

Initial and ongoing assessment assure that the patient is continually being evaluated so that their treatment is specific and relevant to their changing needs. Well designed groups and flexible group leaders guarantee a structure that is perceived as stable, while being responsive to the unique needs of each patient.

The Geriatric Therapeutic Activities staff distinct contribution in clinical rounds has impacted upon all disciplines planning for treatment, family therapy and discharge. The patients report valuing the program because it gives them the varied opportunities and support they need to meet the challenges of growing older with dignity and purpose.

REFERENCES

Cumming, E., Henry, W. (1961). *Growing old: the process of disengagement.* New York: Basic Books.

Fidler, G.S. (1984). *Design of rehabilitation services in psychiatric hospital settings.* Laurel, MD: RAMSCO Publishing.

Gurland, B., Golden, R.G., Teresi, J.A., Challop, J. (1984). The SHORT—CARE: An efficient instrument for the assessment of depression, dementia and disability. *Journal of Gerontology,* Vol. 39, No. 2, pp. 166-169.

Havighurst, R.J. (1961). Successful aging. *Gerontologist,* Vol. 1, pp. 8-13.

Havighurst, R.J., Neugarten, B.L., Tobin, S.S. (1968). Disengagement and patterns of aging. In B.L. Neugarten (Ed.) *Middle age and aging,* Illinois: University of Chicago Press, pp. 161-172.

Maddox, G.L. (1965). Fact and artifact: evidence bearing on the disengagement theory from the Duke Geriatrics Project. *Human Development,* Vol. 8, pp. 117-130.

Mosey, A.C. (1970). *Three frames of reference for mental health.* New Jersey: Charles B. Slack, Inc.

Pikunas, J. (1969). *Human development: an emergent science.* New York: McGraw Hill.

Smith, J.J., Lipman, A. (1972). Constraint and life satisfaction. *Journal of Gerontology,* pp. 77-82.

Weiner, M.B., Brok, A.J., Snadowsky, A.M. (1978). *Working with the aged.* New Jersey: Prentice-Hall, Inc.